D0728638

Date: 6/6/16

616.0472 SOL
Solomon, Kathilyn, 1959-
Tapping into wellness :using EFT
to clear emotional & physical pain

PALM BEACH COUNTY
LIBRARY SYSTEM
3650 SUMMIT BLVD.
WEST PALM BEACH, FL 33406

Praise for *Tapping Into Wellness*

"*Tapping Into Wellness* is for anyone who wants to get to a more empowered place in life. Whether you suffer from stress, overwhelm, or that annoying sabotage behavior, you can get well again using EFT. Thank you Kathilyn for such a comprehensive description and how-to guide for using EFT for the most common challenges that get in our way of being our best selves."

—Carol Look, LCSW, EFT Master, author of *Attracting Abundance with EFT* and *The Tapping Diet,* www.carollook.com

"An excellent resource for you to tap into the rich treasure of your mind-body system and release your fears, resolve your past traumas, heal your sicknesses, and far more ... This book is a fabulous and engaging read, and highly recommended."

—Eric B. Robins, MD and mind-body healing expert, co-author of *Your Hands Can Heal You*

"*Tapping Into Wellness* is an excellent resource for anyone wishing to move beyond the troubling thoughts and feelings that limit their experience of life."

—Brad Yates, author of *Freedom at Your Fingertips* and featured expert in *The Tapping Solution*

"A fantastic primary resource for learning the practical no nonsense EFT ... [that] guides any newcomer to EFT through a succinct way to achieve results quickly and easily."

—Alina Frank, Matrix Reimprinting trainer and mentor at EFT Tapping Training

"*Tapping Into Wellness* will be a rich resource for you: clear information, helpful suggestions and thoughtful tapping strategies that will shine a light of hope into dark corners."

—Rue Ann Hass, MA, EFT Master and Spiritual Life Path Coach

"[*Tapping Into Wellness*] guides you clearly, step by step, to address the issue, dissolve your problems, and transform your life. Genuine, positive, encouraging, this is a book you'll turn to again and again."

—Reneé Marshall Brown, EFT Practitioner, Intuitive Healing and Personal Development Master, and author of the CD *Songs of the Soul*

"Kathilyn's refreshingly honest, compassionate, and caring style is a comforting guide for people ready to make bold and meaningful life changes using this remarkable set of modern day techniques."

—Jondi Whitis, EFT Master Trainer & Trainer of Trainers,
AAMET International, and founder of the Tapfest Spring Energy Event

"A quick and simple authoritative guide to addressing the problems and nagging patterns in your life."

—Karin Davidson, EFT trainer and mentor, AMT EFT Master,
co-author of Level 1-3 EFT coursebooks, and President of
Alternative and Comprehensive Healthcare Professionals

"Laden with meaning about the things that really matter, her book both artfully and clearly communicates her message. It is a delight to read and very easy to digest."

—Rita Davern, parent educator, filmmaker

"[*Tapping Into Wellness*] will lead you by the hand, answer your questions, and provide insights into the workings of the mind."

—Ruthi Backenroth, Matrix Reimprinting and
Advanced EFT Practitioner

TAPPING INTO WELLNESS

About the Author

Kathilyn Solomon delights in, rejoices in, and is nourished by wholehearted, whole-body participation in and sharing of the healing, creative, and errtthy-wrrx-based arts. She is certified or expert in various holistic modalities, including as an AAMET EFT advanced practitioner, as an ACEP ACP-EFT practitioner, as tapping teacher and mentor, as a Faster EFT Level 2 practitioner, creative coach, and herbalist/gardener. In addition to her tapping practice, she also works as a writer, editor, and content queen. She is the mother of Solomon Kasper Probosz, aka Sol. *Tapping Into Wellness* is her eighth book, but her first in the healing arena. For more information, visit her website at www.EFTMinnesota.com.

To Write to the Author

If you wish to contact the author or would like more information about this book, please write to the author in care of Llewellyn Worldwide Ltd. and we will forward your request. Both the author and publisher appreciate hearing from you and learning of your enjoyment of this book and how it has helped you. Llewellyn Worldwide Ltd. cannot guarantee that every letter written to the author can be answered, but all will be forwarded. Please write to:

Kathilyn Solomon
℅ Llewellyn Worldwide
2143 Wooddale Drive
Woodbury, MN 55125-2989

Please enclose a self-addressed stamped envelope for reply, or $1.00 to cover costs. If outside the U.S.A., enclose an international postal reply coupon.

Many of Llewellyn's authors have websites with additional information and resources. For more information, please visit our website at http://www.llewellyn.com.

KATHILYN SOLOMON

TAPPING INTO WELLNESS

Using EFT to Clear Emotional & Physical Pain & Illness

Llewellyn Publications
Woodbury, Minnesota

Tapping Into Wellness: Using EFT to Clear Emotional & Physical Pain & Illness © 2015 by Kathilyn Solomon. All rights reserved. No part of this book may be used or reproduced in any manner whatsoever, including Internet usage, without written permission from Llewellyn Publications, except in the case of brief quotations embodied in critical articles and reviews.

FIRST EDITION
First Printing, 2015

Cover design by Kevin R. Brown
Cover illustration by Jesse Reisch/Deborah Wolfe LTD

Llewellyn is a registered trademark of Llewellyn Worldwide Ltd.

Library of Congress Cataloging-in-Publication Data
Solomon, Kathilyn, 1959–
Tapping into wellness : use EFT to clear emotional & physical pain & illness / Kathilyn Solomon. — First edition.
pages cm
Includes bibliographical references.
ISBN 978-0-7387-3788-1
1. Pain—Alternative treatment. 2. Mental healing. 3. Emotion-focused therapy. I. Title.
RB127.S655 2015
616'.0472—dc23
2015030273

Llewellyn Worldwide Ltd. does not participate in, endorse, or have any authority or responsibility concerning private business transactions between our authors and the public.

All mail addressed to the author is forwarded but the publisher cannot, unless specifically instructed by the author, give out an address or phone number.

Any Internet references contained in this work are current at publication time, but the publisher cannot guarantee that a specific location will continue to be maintained. Please refer to the publisher's website for links to authors' websites and other sources.

Llewellyn Publications
A Division of Llewellyn Worldwide Ltd.
2143 Wooddale Drive
Woodbury, MN 55125-2989
www.llewellyn.com

Printed in the United States of America

Disclaimer

The case studies and stories are based on clients, colleagues, family members, or friends of the author who have given legal permission to have their stories here. Names and case features have been adapted to protect privacy.

Emotional Freedom Techniques (EFT) has produced remarkable clinical results. While scientific evidence indicates EFT's promise as a treatment for a number of conditions, tapping must be considered in the experimental stage. Nothing herein must be construed as guaranteeing or promising benefits or results or as dispensing medical or professional advice.

If you are under the care of a medical or mental health professional, consult your healthcare professional prior to using the techniques and procedures described herein. You, the reader, take full responsibility for using this technique. The author may not be held liable in any way for any loss or damages caused or alleged to be caused directly or indirectly from use of this book's contents.

The author refers to EFT and Gold Standard EFT™ developed by Gary Craig, but this book is not sponsored or endorsed by him. The author is grateful to Gary Craig for his generosity, openheartedness, and tireless efforts to bring EFT/Gold Standard EFT™, Official EFT™, and Optimal EFT™ to the world in an affordable, accessible manner—with integrity.

Dedication

To my son, sweet, beautiful Sol, all grown up now. Being entrusted with the divine gift of raising you, being your Mama, has been the deepest, most enriching, transformative, and just plain good part of my life. Thanks for abiding with maturity beyond your years all the *sturm und drang* involved in birthing this book. You have certainly benefited from a tapping Mama.

To the single parents. To the orphans. To the ones who mistakenly believe that they are the tough cases, to those who are convinced that they can't heal or that they dare not be seen. To the ones who believe they are unlovable or that it may work for others but not for themselves. Or that it's not safe. To the ones who have misplaced their hope. Here now is the time to uncover what's always been there, your amazing self, glorious beyond measure. May this book help you restore what you believe had been lost.

And last but not in the least, to my mother, Lois Clare Solomon, for listening, seeing me, and supporting me, and to my late beloved father, Jerome Sidney Solomon, aka Yos, without whom I would not be.

Contents

Exercises

Acknowledgments

Thanks, in no particular order, to the following: Rita Davern, for listening all those times with an open heart. Thank you for helping me empty the bucket. Kevin Conley, Lady's Champion, game for most everything, including the outrageous lengths I go to for a laugh, with you as prop. Reneé Brown, for spiritual midwifery, working with me regularly on the *you know what,* for introducing me to EFT, and for all the "You Go Grrl's!"

Jondi Whitis, for your generosity and enthusiasm, editorial and tapping work, perspective, and last-minute cutting. For my beloved Mama, Lois Clare—they don't make models like you anymore!—and for your support, love, encouragement, and belief in your number four daughter and her dreams. Matthew Wood, author, half-Jew, half-Indian, half-bear, whole wizard spiritual warrior, wholehearted herbalist extraordinaire—you received a mumbo-jumbo text and opened your home for the writing space, no questions asked. Clare's Well, you are deeply missed, Sisters, but live on in my heart. Peggy Henrikson, for hanging in there, encouragement, upbeat presence, and copy-editorial acumen, making the book look good. For the three who came before me: Barbara "Solomon Optical," for your count-on-ability, your sweet nature, generosity, know-how, grounding, and authority—and for the glasses! Maggie, for answering my call to help without question more than a few times, and for the amazing car, and love. Sandy, for your deep presence and persistence, your beauty inside and out, and for your art infused in all you do and who you are.

Weber, Hoyt, and Hansen families, sisters Barbara and Maggie, and John Howard, you time and again opened your hearts and homes to Sol and me when I needed to be away. My clients, you have taught me much, deeply inspired me, and entrusted me with your tender hearts and stories. I am honored to partner with you in this healing process. I am the lucky one who gets to see you uncover and make manifest the glorious treasure of your essence that is always there under the hurts. To witness the transformation that forgiveness and peace bring is to drink the draught from the eternal well of love and life. Your successes believed me in my own abilities and fed confidence. Those who reviewed chapters gave invaluable feedback: Melody S., David B., Joyce G., Kari T., Barb, and many, many more.

To friends: Ruthi Backenroth, colleague and wise woman, master line editrix and practitioner, and tapping buddy. Ruthi Sloven, adopted sista, it's rare to have so much red-white-and blue powerhouse of love, dance, song, wisdom, spirit, and editorial acumen in one four-foot-something woman! Tasha Tashee, wolf woman, for your care—you brought me back to center—and to cheesecake—more than once. Mr. Purr, for your snuggles and for modeling relaxation. Cougar, you rock! Shannon Pennefeather—thanks for making this connection!

Thanks to the healers and teachers who spurred this work forward, named and unnamed, including the late Suzanne Rivers, you were right about movement for me, the late Gilbert Walking Bull, Laura Morning Star, Rebecca Bradshaw, Tara Brach, Josh Korda, Piotr. To those who held the space for me and my dreams when I forgot and fell into a hole. You reached out your hands, opened your hearts, and slaked my spirit's thirst: Kathleen Zucker-Ducker, Marda K, Jill Strunk, Bill Torvund, Katherine Krumweide (to notre santé!), Kim Hart, curandisma and facilitator of the restoration of the inner Goddess, Amy New Neighbor S., Cecilia Bartok S., Cecilia R., Patricia W., Robert S., Alan C., Ken B., Abby, Tiff and Jean, the Interplay people and process, and more. Gary Craig, for your care and time, for answering the phone (!) and my questions, for discussing this project with me, and encouraging me toward Gold Standard EFT. For Hebrew, glorious, life-giving sacred language of creation, you inspired me throughin and throughout. For the Llewellyn people: Cheryl, you waited and held the door and copy machine open for me! Acquiring editor Angela Wix, your gentleness, patience, structural clarity, availability, and encouragement are a source of reassurance and support. You rode this through to completion and believed in me. Production editor Laura Graves, for making the moving and sometimes messy parts work together, and for your patience with the handwritten final changes. As well, to those not named, those who cannot be named, those I inadvertently forgot, those seen and unseen who helped me own this project and bring this long-overdue baby to birth. I am grateful. I am great-full! Thank you!

Introduction
to Emotional Freedom Techniques

Do you have a problem you can't solve? Are you caught in the grip of a bad memory? Having trouble handling conflict without freaking out? Can't say no? Do you go into fight-or-flight mode each time the boss emails, or have a sex life that is absent without official leave, or food cravings that have gone off the rails? Do you suffer from a serious illness or chronic pain, or from a twenty-first-century lifestyle that fills you with stress and anxiety? Emotional Freedom Technique (aka EFT, tapping, energy therapy, meridian therapy) is a simple practice that can help you address your concerns and offer relief.

What Is EFT and How Might It Help You?

So what exactly *is* EFT? Is tapping talk therapy? No, though talking is involved. Is it acupuncture? No, though you do tap gently on acupressure points. Does it look weird? Perhaps, but no more weird than a Zumba class or acupuncture session to the uninitiated. Is it hard to learn? Absolutely not. Children can easily learn and use it.

EFT is part of a fast-growing area of healing and self-improvement called energy therapy developed by Gary Craig. It regularly gives people long-lasting, permanent relief from bothersome emotional, physical, or performance-related problems. Gold Standard EFT helps clear at the roots deep-seated issues that have caused trouble and upset for years. The process involves you simply holding the thoughts, feelings, and body sensations associated with a targeted problem in mind while tapping on calming points on the upper body. Since its development in 1995, EFT's growth has been exponential; millions worldwide draw on it as a tool to relieve stresses and trauma daily. I've used EFT to relieve bad memories and trauma, stress, anxiety, self-sabotage, and much more. I've tapped on the emotional components, bad memories and experiences, and physical symptoms relating to a physical pain, illness, or disease and witnessed remarkably, the physical problems resolve, from fibromyalgia to phantom limb pain. I've used tapping to stop bleeding on someone after a traumatic fall. I've used it with toddlers to resolve separation anxiety, terror and tantrums, and other upsets, and on parents to resolve lacking confidence and feelings of failure as moms and dads. I've used it with entrepeneurs as well as those who are stuck to unstick and joyfully move onto the next level of their lives and successes. I've used it to help people overcome performance-related issues, including professional athletes who cleared out difficulties getting back in the game after an accident. I've used it to stop pain, improve sleep, resolve cravings, raise self esteem and confidence, and to simply access a more wholesome, peaceful, and connected way of experiencing the world. Really, I've tried it on just about anything and everyone—including my cat, Mr. Purr.

Tapping works with all parts of you—your feelings, your body sensations, your conscious and subconscious mind, and your body's energy system to help resolve trauma. I also believe it works on "a quantum level," let's call it. (Interestingly, EFT and Gold Standard Founder Gary Craig is now exploring the spiritual nature of tapping, with much of his work not involving tapping at all).Your whole self participates to release the grip the problem has on you and the grip you have on a problem, which can allow you to experience relief on a number of levels—physical, emotional, performance-related, and spiritual.

The therapeutic field is beginning to appreciate the importance of body procedures and energy therapy in relation to healing traumatic experiences, too.[1] Scientific studies indicate tapping's effectiveness in treating many different psychological disorders.[2] A growing number of therapists and medical professionals, teachers and business leaders, and others in diverse industries, use tapping to benefit their work in everything from hospitals and clinics to schools and corporations and more. It's even being introduced in to some graduate psychology courses.

EFT restores your ability to think clearly, to experience a sense of wellbeing, and to feel good again, no matter your circumstances. Whether you have a physical problem, emotional upset, or performance issue, EFT can become your own personal self-applied problem zapper. It aims a laser-beam focus at a difficult feeling or thought, problem, situation, or memory, and neutralizes it. While there is no guarantee that tapping will resolve a physical ailment, people regularly experience relief from physical symptoms after collapsing the emotional factors and other events underlying physical challenges. It's free, easy to learn, self-applied, safe, and can be done anywhere, at any time, on any issue, on people of all ages (including four-legged "people"). I've seen EFT save jobs, friendships, health, marriages, and sanity. Even if you don't believe tapping will work for you, it can help—and quickly, as you'll see in examples throughout this book. EFT opens windows that have been painted shut for years,

---

1. Peter Levine, PhD, developer of Somatic Experiencing®; "Getting to the Root of Trauma," (Podcast talk in *Rethinking Trauma* Series hosted by Ruth M. Buczynski, PhD.), Accessed November 18, 2014, www.nicabm.com/treating- trauma2014/post-info/.

2. David Feinstein, PhD, "Acupoint Stimulation In Treating Psychological Disorders: Evidence of Efficacy." *Review of General Psychology* Vol. 16 (4), 364–380. Accessed January 15, 15. doi:10.1037/a0028602.

letting fresh air in. It helps close doors on difficult chapters of your life that have been propped open, letting all kinds of riff-raff in, and it gives you tools to clear out the dusty nooks and crannies of your life. It is about changing your thinking so you can change your life. EFT releases the charge around the bad memories; the limiting beliefs and thoughts, and it restores your energy system to balance, giving you a clean slate. It's empowering. It's free. Its applications are pretty much infinite. With this book as your guide, you'll start tapping on the challenges that come along. You'll know how to systematically neutralize bad memories, fears, and limiting beliefs; and you'll clearly understand the process and the tools you can access depending on your tapping target. You will feel better. I can attest to that!

How I Came to EFT

I was in the East Village of Manhattan, working in publishing, as an author and editor. I was very good but even better at turning down amazing career offers. I had a deep-seated belief: "I'm not good enough," and though clearly the reality was different, I went with the old, "safe" belief. Eventually I left publishing altogether driven in part by the stress of insecurity and fear of getting things wrong, and other mind-bending lies. I had plenty of limiting beliefs, core issues, and self-sabotage—not that I understood it that way back then. Fast-forward a few years: I was nine months pregnant and due any day, writing for a medical school with an avocation as an herbalist, in deep denial about my long unhappy marriage. I was expecting to birth my baby at home, and my seven-page birth plan was truly a work of art. Its indications—for lavender massage oil, hand-made tinctures, electrolytes, specific directions to my birth support team, Gyuto monks chanting for opening the birthway passage—anticipated everything, almost.

A near-death experience wasn't part of the plan. Due to labor and delivery complications, my newborn son experienced fetal distress and birth trauma, and I bled profusely just after he was born.

To truly love, one must open, and my beloved, long-awaited son's birth opened doors of denial that had been long closed. They burst open, no going back. Years of unprocessed and unresolved emotional experiences bubbled up. In my weakened physical state, I who had made sure to never need anyone, suddenly needed help everywhere. My mind body and spirit simply could not handle everything all at once. In a weakened state, my recovery faltered and then shut down as fear ramped up. The marriage ended like an amputation, just that suddenly, and the loss of my health, money, status (an illusion anyway), friends, and worldly goods came swiftly. Post-traumatic stress syndrome, liver trauma, postpartum depression, fibromyalgia, took up residence, but I had my now toddler son and my life. In those years, my inner critic or negative thoughts galloped along paths like these and I believed these lies: *I can't do this. I am guilty for leaving my son's dad. I am a burden. What a loser! They don't like me. I don't belong. This is too hard.* My beliefs may have echoed those of other family members, including those in my lineage.

The compulsive self-talk did not help my situation. Rather than acknowledging my strengths—my courage, compassion, creativity, resourcefulness, persistence and determination, fierce loving nature—I focused on how "bad" I was—my shame ruled. I believed mothers couldn't relate to me, and I didn't blame them. Such stories I made up in my brilliant, active, creative mind! As if any of us are really anything other than connected in our very essence.

Fibromyalgia is an illness for which Western medicine has no cure; I had no belief in my ability to heal, and it set me back. The pain was debilitating. I hurt all the time. Like other autoimmune illnesses, fibromyalgia is invisible. You can't see it the way you can a rash or cast on a broken leg. To many, people with autoimmune illnesses seem like slackers.

While I was careening downhill, many hands reached out to catch my fall, including those of: Sister Maria, of blessed memory, my family, a few wise women friends, and Reneé Brown, an intuitive healer and teacher. She introduced me to EFT, commonly called tapping. Amazingly, when I tapped, I felt better.

All I did was think of a troubling issue and come up with a number from 0 to 10 to measure how badly the problem bothered me right at that moment. Then I focused on that problem while tapping on stress-reducing points on my upper body and saying an affirmation that I accepted myself. It was that simple; I didn't even have to believe that I accepted myself, that I loved myself, or that I forgave myself—which was a good thing, because I damn well wasn't going to forgive myself for the mess I'd gotten myself into at that time (that came later). I listened to and tapped along with Gary Craig's training DVDs (See EFT Resources for details) even when it was time for bed I'd turn them on and listen in my sleep.

Holes started appearing in my misery and hopelessness, letting light flood in. Outwardly, my life appeared the same, but my inner world began to change. I began to see things differently. I understood now I wasn't shameful or bad. I was just experiencing a different life than the one I had expected and different from many other people I knew (definitely not life on the surface!) This was and is a life that was deepening me, carving beautiful wisdom, expanding my ability to love and have compassion for others, driving me to transform unhealthy family and cultural parenting patterns, and helping me understand how truly glorious I and every other human being with whom I came into contact is, was, and always will be. I I realized I was a very loving and good mom; I had many, many beings, seen and unseen, who loved me and supported me, and I had good fortune beyond what I could even fathom The pain began to subside. Life began to change for the better.

At "EFT for Serious Diseases," the first of many workshops I along with hundreds of others attended that featured Gary Craig and other EFT masters sharing teaching and working with people onstage, I witnessed people experiencing relief from serious emotional trauma and/or physical symptoms. They experienced profound emotional breakthroughs and insights, and so did I, tapping along with everyone else in the audience. We "borrowed benefits," receiving results on our own issues, because that's how EFT works. Like Mother Nature, tapping indiscriminately showers healing.

I witnessed people's harmful cravings and addictions dissolve. The issue wasn't the craving, but the underlying unmet needs, forgotten or fiercely remembered traumatic memories (and sometimes forgotten good memories), limiting beliefs, distorted perceptions, and outgrown coping mechanisms. Then, my fibromyalgia eased, and finally disappeared. Am I done healing? You may as well ask if I'm done learning. Everyday is an opportunity and a choice to grow, learn, heal, love, and to stay connected with what really matters—the truth beyond what we see with our eyes. About that experience I had so long ago, when I "lost" everything? Actually, that was the divine opportunity for me to deeply connect with who I am; to learn how to experience true intimacy; to embody the fierce love of a mother toward the holy being entrusted to her care—my amazing, glorious, ever surprising son with whom I enjoy a loving, joyful, alive, and flowing deep nourishing river of a relationship; and to have the compassion, understanding, and acceptance to sit with others in their pain and help them help themselves in my EFT practice. The door that busted open after my son's birth was the biggest blessing of my life. No way would I have given all that other stuff that seemed so real up without a near death experience! I have a teaching practice—not just EFT—and have resumed my writing and editorial business in a way that works also for me. Along with a life that continues laden with possibilities. It keeps getting better, as I continue to remember that it's all about connection—first with Self, then with others, and my belief, that we are all, at heart, one.

In addition to the certifications of completion and certifications I earned early on in association with Gary Craig's early EFT work, I am one of a small number of EFT practitioners who has earned the Association for Comprehensive Energy Psychology's (ACEP) ACP-EFT practitioner credential, under the direction, mentorship, and extensive training of Tina Craig in the use of Gold Standard EFT. I also have earned AAMET (Association for the Advancement of Meridian Energy Techniques) International's Advanced Practitioner credential. I teach and offer demos and workshops and ongoing groups on tapping. Additional body, mind, and spirit-enhancing practices that support my healthy work and life include Ayurvedic daily routine, western hands-on herbalism and medicine-making, Neuro-linguistic Programming (NLP), study of many varied interests, including brain development and memory reconsolidation, emerging forms of tapping, inspiring thought-leaders, meditation, yoga, exercise, dance, interplay, social joy, parenting by connection, daily spiritual practice including gratitudes, and more, including and especially play.

I'm blessed with clients who show me how resilient the human spirit is, demonstrating the possibility of healing from even the darkest of places. And I believe in their ability to heal, as I do yours, because I've witnessed it in so many others and in myself.

What we think of as bad doesn't need to sideline us. If we can just make a little room for all of us to surround even the yucky parts with love, we heal. Emotion is not something we should fear. Emotion or feelings, are the stuff of life, in all their glory, subtlety, and variations. May they come to be embraced and accepted just as the colors and melodies of our universe. Emotional Freedom is a wondrous thing. It allows a person to own her life. Did I hear you ask: Was I scared to write this book? You might say I had a lot of opportunities to tap and address old, old fears. Of course, that was along with a great deal of excitement and joy at this opportunity to share my learning and this profound technique. And I kept on writing right through the fears. I did it for me—that's called courage—and for you—because EFT has much to offer. You'll soon see.

What You Will Find in This Book

The approach in this book is largely based on Gold Standard EFT tapping, which means it offers specified, consistent techniques and standards that show how to find, aim at, and manage a tapping target and get at the roots underlying a presenting today issue. It is a technique that consistently gets results. In this book, your path to emotional freedom is laid out in two parts: Part I shows the nuts and bolts of EFT tapping, and Part II shows how to apply EFT to specific, common situations and conditions. A Resources section and Appendices offer additional information at the book's end. The text is clear, laden with easy-to-follow tapping exercises and interesting case studies to demonstrate different issues that can come up during a tapping session and how to find your way through them to resolution. Once you know the Gold Standard basics of tapping, you can really jump in anywhere. An exercise list makes it easy to find exercises according to topic. However, this isn't a sprint, it's a marathon. Healing is a process. You can take your time. Have a notebook so you can follow the exercises, note insights, and track progress. This will be your EFT journal to use and return to over time. And you can use this book as a reference time and again, as needed. May you experience blessings a thousandfold in your life as a result of your life's learning. Enjoy, from here forward, the integration of EFT into your life.

PART I
Getting Started with EFT

Part I includes chapters 1 through 5. Chapter 1 covers the history and development of EFT and meridian tapping, how EFT works and why it is so effective, the science behind tapping, and hands-on one-point tapping to get you started. Chapter 2 shows you how to tap using the Gold Standard EFT basic recipe. By the end of this chapter you'll know how to tap and will have tried tapping on specific events. Chapter 3 shows you how to get specific and practical with EFT to get results and what to watch for when you are not getting the changes you seek. You'll access the EFT workhorse tools such as Tell the Story and Personal Peace Procedure in chapter 4, going further into tapping techniques that you can apply systematically to obtain relief from bad memories, fears and other troubling feelings, unfortunate habits and behaviors, and difficult negative self-talk and belief systems. Chapter 5 offers practical tips and tricks, as well as answers to commonly asked questions, including how to find a trustworthy practitioner. Got your EFT journal handy? Let's get started.

Chapter 1

Introducing Emotional Freedom Techniques, or EFT

I was making tea in the kitchen when it happened. I had just lifted the full four-quart pot of boiling water off the stove and was about to pour it into the teapot when I dropped the pan. Boiling hot water immediately saturated the heel, toes, and sole of the sock on my left foot and began traveling up the ankle. The pain seared deep into my foot. I gasped for my friend to come and help. Pain had taken my breath away.

Finally, I got my tight knee-high sock off. Pink burns colored the bottom and sides of my foot. The pain was unbearable! However, when my friend suggested icing my foot and going to the ER, I shook my head no—I was literally unable to speak—and applied EFT tapping. I was sure EFT would work—and at the same time, not sure at all. I hated the idea of going to the ER, however, and ice felt like an interruption.

I tapped the EFT points on my upper body continuously as I experienced what was happening *right now.* I kept tapping the calming points, whimpering all the while. After a couple minutes, I caught my breath enough that I could now speak. The pain was about a 10, on the pain scale. I spoke out loud while tapping on the first EFT point on the side of my hand, the Karate Chop point: "Even though this really really really hurts, I deeply and completely accept myself!" I tapped on phrases like, "Oww! Oww! Oww!," and "I can't believe I did this!"

I tapped on the surprise and shock, on the fear I wouldn't be able to walk, and on the concern I'd need to cancel an upcoming EFT training. Then I returned to tapping on the sensations, the feelings, and the other thoughts stemming from the burn event. Suddenly, I realized the pain was gone. Maybe fifteen or twenty minutes had passed. My friend was open-mouthed in disbelief. And that was that.

A burn that should have put me in the emergency room was completely gone except for a few little pink streaks that didn't even look like burns. Once again, I was blown away by the fact that EFT had worked.

Tapping on the feelings of pain had literally whooshed the sensations through and out of my body, giving my immune system the ability to do its job without being handicapped by the additional onslaught of stressful emotions, limiting beliefs, and negative self-talk. But how had tapping resulted in healing of my burned foot? What the tapping did was focus me and my body's energy system on the sensations, feelings, beliefs, and thoughts relating to the experience. I was immersed in all of my emotions about the event while tapping on them. Had I not tapped, I would have gone to the ER, had blisters, taken a while to heal, and wouldn't have been able to lead training. I experienced relief instead.

Simple—Try It on Everything—Everyone Can Do It

The EFT process itself is elegantly simple, and you'll know how to apply it for yourself by the end of chapter 2. You tap gently with your fingertips on naturally calming points on your body while focused, as in the previous example, on a troubling event and its associated feelings, sensations, and thoughts. Tapping helps your body's energy system rebalance. You experience relief from that particular upset that is long-term and often permanent. It's not magic, however.

Tapping about your divorce or bankruptcy won't cause you to be happily married or financially solvent. It will allow you to have peace and well-being, even as you think about the problem. It can help you see and understand what you could not see or understand before when thinking was clouded with emotion or protection mechanisms were preventing you from seeing the truth.

Interestingly, when you tap on one problem of today or a past memory and it resolves, other areas of your life sometimes completely unrelated may also change for the better. For example, clearing the memory of a parent who said you'll never amount to anything may surprise you in that your right hip pain resolves or a great career opportunity suddenly opens up and you suddenly really understand and forgive your parent, who was doing the best he or she could.

One at a time, you can effectively break down the really big issues into bite-size, solvable chunks. As you grow in this process, avalanches of sabotaging behaviors, stresses, anxieties, health issues or physical problems, and performance issues can simply collapse. Even the stuff you thought you'd never change can change. In this book, you'll see the tough stuff people have overcome with tapping. An added bonus is that you begin to have more forgiveness and acceptance of others.

EFT and Trauma: The Light, the Candle, or the Circuit Breaker?

When we have an upset that we experience as traumatic, the body's energy system literally short-circuits. We call this an "energy disruption" in EFT. When this happens, we have difficult feelings, and we are unable to digest, understand, and move through and beyond an unpleasant experience. And anytime we remember the "bad" experience or when something reminds us of it, even if the memory was from a long time ago, we experience the disruption again.

Imagine a lamp that suddenly goes dark. The light bulbs and lamp seem fine, yet the light doesn't work. We may adjust by using candles, but the candle burns down, leaving us in darkness. This is the equivalent of merely coping to survive. But what if the problem is simply a blown fuse in the central circuit breaker box? All you need to do is flip the circuit breaker switch back to on, and the lamp will work again. Surprisingly, our body-mind is not so different.

When we experience what our body-mind believes to be an assault on our survival, our body's energy system shifts to survival mode. We experience what EFT calls an energy disruption, a disconnect in the flow of our energy, or a zzzt! Think of a cat with its fur on end as analogous to what your energy system does when it is disrupted. The result? Negative emotions and rumination, compulsions, painful symptoms, phobias, allergies, self-sabotage, and other unhelpful behaviors. And we go as far as we can to avoid this situation altogether or anything that remotely resembles the original painful upset.

When we experience an event as traumatic, we go into survival mode, and we're cut off from the part of our brain responsible for mature, reasoned, insightful thinking called the neocortex. Instead, we are in an adrenalized state of being, commonly known as fight-flight-or-freeze, in which there's no room for thinking things through and feeling our feelings. The brain stem, that primitive and reptilian part of our brain, is in charge now. In this state of being, the amygdala, a small almond-shaped part of your brain's limbic system, says in its own language: "Ohmygosh! Danger danger danger! We're all gonna die! Save us!" The amygdala instantaneously communicates this emergency alert to the body. The heart races and adrenal glands start working to give us superhuman strength; digestive action and all other noncritical bodily functions are put on hold as we act like the gazelle that instinctively flees the tiger.

In traumatic events, emotions are irrelevant. None of us would have survived if our ancestors had taken the time to explore their feelings about predators chasing them instead of running for their lives. Today, many generations later, we're still hardwired that way.

You may survive a trauma—in this case, a difficult event or experience—but you haven't processed the "e-motions" (think of it as short for "energy in motion") or feelings surrounding the experience. They are stored in your body's sensate memory and in your subconscious mind so you no longer have the conscious ability to feel them. When memories are buried alive, they live on and on inside our psyches. The traumatic experience is stored in the area that holds long-term memory: the limbic brain. When the limbic brain senses that whatever situation you are in is remotely similar to the initial alleged threat, you involuntarily launch into survival mode.

Have you ever overreacted to something out of proportion to the situation but couldn't help it? Ever acted against your own best interests or irrationally? You may be touching on a buried traumatic event. When triggered, it's like falling through a trapdoor. These booby traps are our "distress patterns," our energy disruptions, and we all have them. You can go from feeling good and competent to shooting yourself in the foot, sabotaging yourself, or feeling like a worthless mess who can't ever get anything right. Ironically enough, your primitive brain is simply doing its job to keep you safe and on the planet. It's conducting twenty-four-hour surveillance to make sure you stay far away from that experience where you had that initial energy disruption, or circuit break. Here's how that might look:

- Nina regularly copes with stressful days not by acknowledging how painful and difficult they are, but by binge eating, insulating herself. She learned early in her life to assuage painful feelings with comfort food. The food soothes, but only temporarily.

- Normally confident, Bruce gets tongue-tied at the expense of career advancement when certain aggressive colleagues are present at work meetings. Growing up as the youngest in a large family, he consistently experiences "smack downs" when he voices his opinion.
- Fifty-year-old Soren was in a car crash as a teenager, the fallout of which has extended to the point that she cannot drive on highways anymore.

When we aim EFT at problems like these, we resolve them at their roots. We make healthier choices about food, we speak confidently at work, and we drive on the highway with ease because we have worked through the painful experiences that led us to take up the challenging behaviors. Tapping restores our healthy, resourceful state of being. We reclaim our choice and our options—we reclaim our whole selves.

EFT undoes the short circuit or energy disruption experienced in trauma and rebalances and restores harmony in the body's energy system. Let's explore the core principle of EFT, the Discovery Statement: *The cause of all negative emotions is a disruption in the body's energy system.* This means that it's not the actual memory that causes the trauma and discomfort. It's the disruption in the body's energy flow that happens when a person experiences the problem event, which then results in the difficult emotions, trauma, ensuing troubling behaviors such as self-sabotage, phobias, anxiety, fear, and even physical pain symptoms and illness, in many cases.

To resolve the energy disruption and restore your body-mind system to balance, you need to turn the central circuit breaker back on. Talking about the past bad memory won't touch the trauma housed in the primitive, limbic part of the brain. You need to actually go there, to the part of your system in which the energy disruption occurred. Tapping while focused on a specific problem gets us to where the initial *zzzt!* occurred, as clearly as if we were using GPS. We are now at ground zero of the traumatic memory, where we experience the feelings, sensations, thoughts, and any remembered images or upsetting details, that have been buried, release them, release the trauma, and experience relief. We have basically flipped the thinking-feeling switch back to on, moving the signals and symptoms of life-and-death threat through the limbic system, all the way to "I'm safe and sound now."

By eliminating the roller coaster of emotions, EFT co-creates with you a space for insights and perspective that allows you to act from a position of strength and wisdom. It helps you put the past behind you and experience a better future.

Acupuncture Points EFT Uses: Why They Work

The places you tap with EFT are acupuncture points. Each of us has more than four hundred of these acupuncture points located inside the body on energy pathways called meridians. Refer to Figure 1.

Though invisible to the eye, the body's energy pathways flow like rivers. Acupuncture points are like small oases or islands dotted along the meridians, located where the meridians come closest to the surface of the skin, which makes them easier to access.

Twelve primary meridian pathways flow on each side of the body, interconnected thanks to a secondary meridian pathway network. Hundreds of acupuncture points are scattered throughout these pathways. Each primary pathway is associated with a different organ in the body—kidneys, lungs, heart, and so on. Life force energy, or chi, flows through these rivers, or energy pathways (other names for life force are *prana* in Hindi and *ruakh,* meaning wind or divine spirit in Hebrew).

When the life force streams freely, we feel good. Imagine a river like the Nile, feeding and providing vitality to everything around it. However, if any of the pathways are blocked, vital life force energy

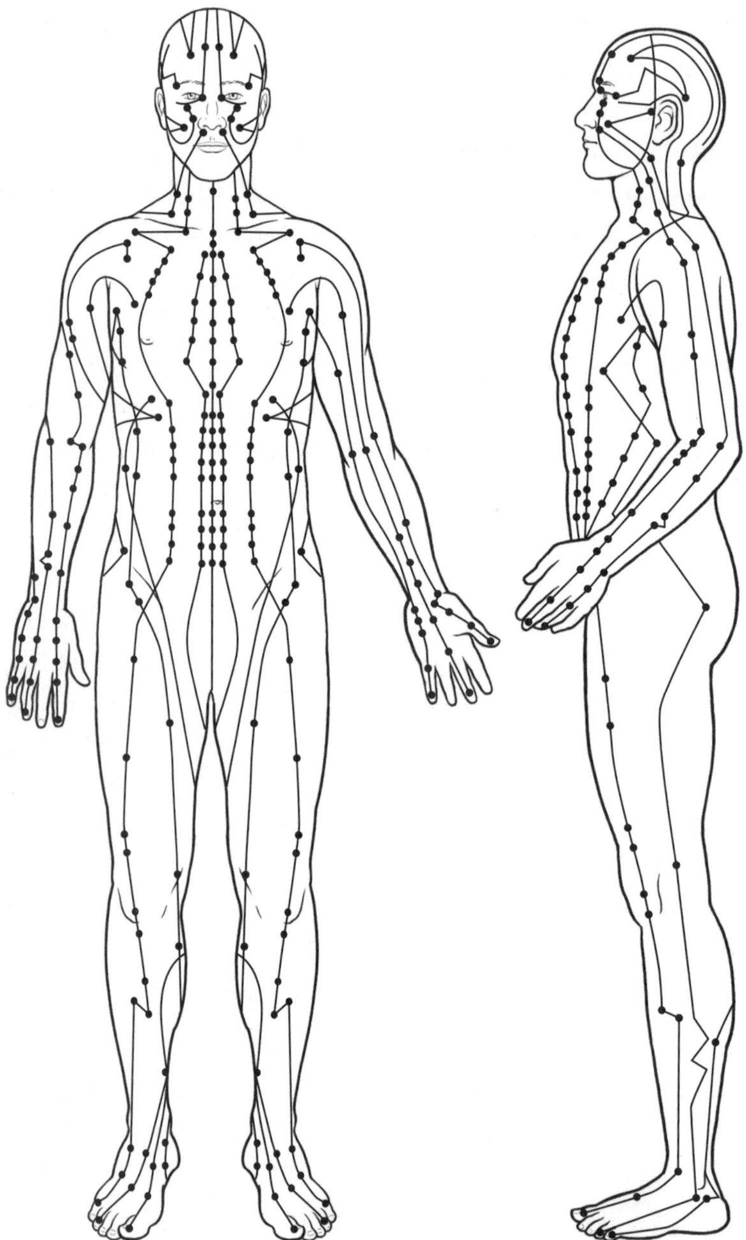

Figure 1: *Twelve principal meridians or pathways flow like rivers of life energy through the body. The tapping points used in EFT are also acupuncture points, situated at points along the meridians nearest to the skin's surface. Tapping on these points moves the most energy.*

can't move freely. We won't feel up to par. If the block remains over time, illness may result.

With acupuncture, needles stimulate our energy system, causing the chi to push through the blockages to restore the flow of life force energy so we experience health. With EFT, we gently tap on the points with our fingertips while mentally focusing on the problem, which initiates a healing response from the body's energy system. The entire process, which has also been described as emotional acupuncture, can unfold quite quickly, facilitating many different feelings or thoughts, shifting body sensation awareness, or bringing about a sudden calm or shift in the way one thinks about a problem. When you tap, you gain an understanding of the whole of what's happening in your body-mind as you focus on one particular target, and it's a profound experience: you're not lost in the problem. Once EFT has resolved your issue, you will no longer obsess about it, feel bad about it, or condemn yourself about it with the same troubling intensity. You might realize that you had the problem and that it used to affect you badly, but you no longer have that issue. You might even acknowledge how good freedom feels and thereby empower yourself even more. Relief! This is how we break the pattern of trauma. Even deep-seated or core issues can be resolved with EFT. That's because the technique itself gets to the core, when applied correctly.

The Science Behind Tapping and Development of EFT

The amount of science demonstrating EFT's effectiveness is growing. The respected American Psychological Association's (APA) journal, *Review of General Psychology,* published an article in 2012 by clinical psychologist Dr. David Feinstein that noted tapping fulfilled the APA standards for being either a "well-established or probably efficacious treatment" for everything from public-speaking issues to phobias, from test-taking anxiety to post-traumatic stress disorder

(PTSD) and depression.[3] Another 2013 study indicated that tapping reduces the level of cortisol, the hormone released when a person feels stress.[4] As of this book's writing, another long-term study is in process offering EFT to veterans who experience post-traumatic stress syndrome (PTSD).

While acupuncture and energy work date back to pretty much the beginning of human history, the roots of EFT began with Thought Field Therapy (TFT), developed by Dr. Roger Callahan, a psychotherapist knowledgeable in both kinesiology and acupuncture. He had a client named Mary who had been terrified of water nearly all her life. She couldn't even take a full bath. One day when Mary mentioned that just thinking of water gave her a terrible feeling in her stomach, Dr. Callahan suggested she tap with her fingers on the acupuncture point related to the stomach, just under the middle of either eye. Within minutes of tapping, Mary leapt from her chair and ran toward the water and dipped her toes in. Her lifelong phobia was gone—for good![5]

Encouraged, Dr. Callahan developed several specific protocols, or tapping sequences, keyed to different acupuncture points to relieve phobia, fear, anger, trauma, and the like. He named this method of energy psychology Thought Field Therapy. A man named Gary Craig was one of those who trained in TFT.

---

3. David Feinstein, Ph.D., "Acupoint stimulation in treating psychological disorders: Evidence of efficacy," *Review of General Psychology,* vol. 16 (4), 364–380, accessed January 15, 2105, doi:10.1037/a0028602.

4. Dawson Church, Ph.D., Grant Young, Ph.D., and Audrey J. Brooks, Ph.D., "The Effect of Emotional Freedom Techniques on Stress Biochemistry: A Randomized Controlled Trial," *The Journal of Nervous and Mental Disease,* Oct. 2012 vol. 200 Issue 10, 891–896, accessed January 11, 2015, journals.lww.com/jonmd/Abstract/2012/10000/The_Effect_of_Emotional_Freedom_Techniques_on.12.aspx.

5. Thought Field Therapy News, "Thirty Years of Thought Field Therapy," Accessed January 11, 2015, www.rogercallahan.com/news/30-years-of-thought-field-therapy/case-studies.

Gary had been an active participant in the self-improvement field for much of his life. He realized that "the quality of [his] thoughts was mirrored in the quality of [his] life." He understood the benefits of TFT. However, TFT training was very costly. Gary, a Stanford-trained engineer who had not actually worked in that field, used his engineer's mind and tinkered with the process and streamlined it, creating a singular technique useful for a wide range of problems, called Emotional Freedom Technique. It worked to resolve both physical and emotional pain as well as performance problems. Even symptoms of serious disease could be resolved when the emotional aspects underlying the illness were addressed.

Gary understood the potential impact that this simple tapping process would have on people everywhere. He began to share EFT (which became Gold Standard EFT later) with as many people as possible, taking tapping on the road, offering trainings, and workshops that were open to everyone.

Around 1998, he released a recording of his work, *6 Days at the VA*, which showed how tapping over six days worked for deeply troubled veterans of the Vietnam War living with severe PTSD. A later film, *The Answer: Operation Emotional Freedom* (2010), documents PTSD-diagnosed vets from Vietnam, Afghanistan, and Iraq conflicts and the profound impact energy psychology had on participants.

Gary started an online newsletter in 1997 that quickly grew to serve a large international online community, with people from around the world sharing their EFT questions, thoughts, case studies, and results. emoFree.com had some 500,000 subscribers at one time, with thousands downloading the original (now obsolete) EFT manual each month.

The evolution of meridian therapy might be considered akin to the explosive development of the World Wide Web; the technology with which it works continues to evolve and surprise us, as is only natural. Gary Craig's contemporaries and students have created other energy therapy protocols or adapted tapping and developed other effective tapping methods. See EFT Resources for more information about these additions.

This book focuses primarily on traditional EFT, which has evolved into the Gold Standard EFT or Official EFT. Gold Standard EFT is the primary, albeit not only, method I draw on in my holistic coaching practice. Occasionally in the text I indicate variations on Gold Standard EFT. The terms "tapping" and "EFT" are used interchangeably.

Please note that I chose to primarily focus on Gold Standard due to the many confusions, variations, and issues raised as a result of inconsistent standards in other tapping variations. This does not mean that other tapping processes do not work, it just means that you will have a solid foundation on which to build your practice. The Gold Standard Program was co-developed by Gary and his daughter, Tina Craig, and directed by Tina thought December of 2015. I have earned the credential and it is the most rigorous, effective, and comprehensive one to date.

Mojo. Juju. Tap. Heal.

No problem is bigger than you are, and no feelings are bigger than you are. You may have experienced traumas in your life that have gotten stuck inside. You may have created solutions to problems that are harder on you and your loved ones than the original problem itself. You may have workarounds to problems or coping mechanisms that no longer work to your benefit. You can use EFT to release the blocks that hold you back.

You can heal, thrive, transform, and feel whole again. You can have your dreams. You can switch up any area of your life with EFT; get back on the road to vibrant health and well-being, reap financial abundance, achieve your goals, enjoy body confidence and loving relationships, and live with peace and tranquility in your heart instead of stress and anxiety.

You can make a difference in your life and in the lives of those around you by learning and practicing EFT. Imagine a small stone thrown into a still pond; ripples expand on the entire surface of water. Consider the effect tapping could have on your world. Can you see how your own peace of mind could change everything?

Getting Started with One-Point Tapping

My tapping clients often express profound surprise and gratitude at the changes they experience in just one tapping session. Tapping gets results fast. Naturally, many clients want to tap on other bad memories and discomforts outside sessions in their daily lives, but some hesitate. They say: "I might get it wrong," "I don't know the right words to say," or "It won't work if I do it on my own." These are known as limiting beliefs, and they are quite common to the condition of being human. The doubts often stretch back to early events in childhood, either consciously remembered or implicit (meaning remembered in the subconscious mind), where the child didn't feel safe.

Here's my response: "There's no failure, only feedback." You can't get tapping wrong, but it won't work if you don't do it!

Even if you're not sure of all the parts of EFT, miss some tapping points, or don't know what to say, you will learn as you go—even if you don't follow the "right" protocol. Most importantly, you'll still get results, because tapping moves energy.

Exercise: One-Point Tapping: A Quick Glimpse

I often start people new to EFT on one tapping point known as the collarbone point. It's a way to get started easily. You're going to learn this now; think of it as EFT on training wheels. One-point tapping uses basic EFT components: identifying an unpleasant feeling or thought, measuring your reaction to it, tapping, and then checking your reaction again to the original unpleasant feeling or thought.

Preparation: Have your EFT journal handy. Notice that no matter where you are, sitting or standing, the earth is rising up to meet and support you. Now, breathe in deeply through your nose, and imagine your breath traveling all the way up through your body, starting with your feet, up your legs, your spine, and out the top of your head, showering up and around your body like an old oak tree canopy. Now, exhale slowly through your mouth, letting it all go. Repeat several times.

Step 1. Identify a mildly unpleasant issue. Allow a mildly unpleasant thought, feeling, or experience to come to mind. If you don't have any, make one up or contact me and I'll share one of mine! When I say "mild troubles or problems," I mean things like "this pain in my right shoulder," "that guy who cut me off in traffic this morning," "the mess my spouse left in the kitchen again," "too much email." Not the big stuff. Select your own little peeve now.

Step 2. Note your intensity rating. How intensely do you feel the upsetting thought, feeling, sensation, or experience you selected? Use a 0 to 10 intensity scale, where 10 is the most intense, upsetting, worst-case scenario feeling and 0 means no upset at all. This is known as the Subjective Units of Distress Scale (SUDS).

Write your intensity rating down in your EFT journal so you won't forget it, as your intensity of feeling will likely change during the exercise. If you don't have a designated notebook or online file, find or create one now. This journal will become your map for navigating through the exercises in this book. You will also use the journal later as a guide and protocol for building your own solid tapping practice.

Step 3. Find the collarbone tapping point. The collarbone point is where the sternum, breastbone, and first rib meet in your body. That little juncture forms a bony U-shape. See Figure 2 for an illustration of the collarbone point location.

The actual points are about an inch down and an inch outward, to the right or left of the collarbone's U bone, not on the bone itself.

You have two points on either side of your collarbone, although we refer to them as a single point.

Now, loosely cup your fingers and thumb and lightly tap all across the top of your chest, like Tarzan. You're tapping on the EFT collarbone points. You can also make a loose fist and thump. Be gentle as you tap, massage, or thump.

Tarzan tap for at least 60 seconds. You are tapping in the area of the thymus gland. The Greek word *thymus* means "life energy."

Step 4. Tuning in and tapping. Now focus on your little peeve or tapping target from step 1, while gently Tarzan tapping the collarbone points. Do this for 60 or more seconds, until the upset subsides, before moving on to the next step.

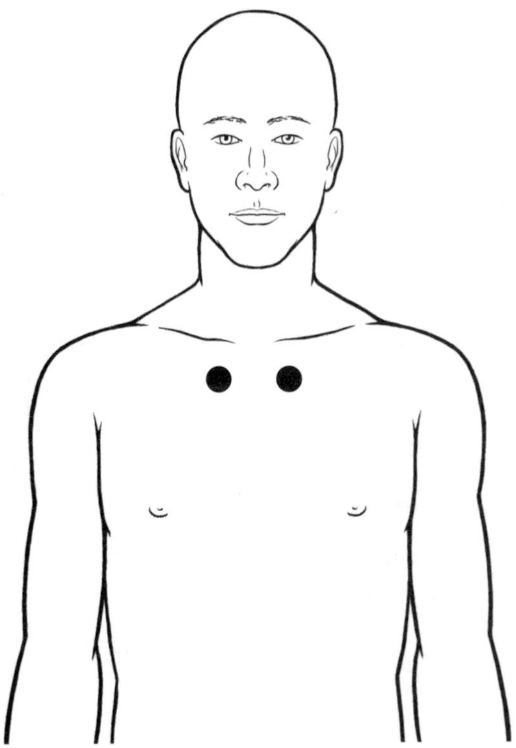

Figure 2: *Thump or tap the collarbone points. These are located on the thymus.*

Step 5. Using a positive phrase. Now imagine that you can set the upset you tapped on aside carefully for the moment (for instance on a comfortable chair or a place where you don't have to keep an eye on it). For 60 seconds or so, continuously Tarzan tap while expressing one or more of the positive thoughts, feelings, images, and beliefs listed below, or make up your own. Speak aloud slowly while tapping:

- *All life tends toward the good.*
- *Peace.*
- *Seeing the colors of sunrise.*
- *Monks chanting.*
- *I appreciate* ______________ (something you appreciate or care about).
- *I choose to release this upset.*
- *Love is the answer.*
- *Sound of babies cooing. Baby soft. Baby fingers.*
- *My life energy is high. I am in the state of love.*[6]
- *Peace, calm, joy, compassion, hope*
- *Courage, grace, love, truth*
- *I'm grateful for my body.*
- *Wow, I love feeling good.*
- *I love how it feels when the sun is shining, and it's not too hot and not too cold, but just right.*
- *Rainbows!*
- *I love* _____ (express a moment from your past where everything was just right).
- *I like waking up feeling refreshed.*
- *Ahhh, the wonderful smell of* ________.
- *The sound of birdsong at sunrise.*

---

6. Dr. John Diamond, MD., Daily Affirmation Program, *Life Energy, Using the Meridians to Unlock the Hidden Power of Your Emotions,* Paragon House, 1990, 219–221.

These thoughts elicit an expansive state of mind which takes one out of the fight-flight-or-freeze adrenalized state.

Step 6. Checking in. Now, check back in on the little peeve or tapping target you initially identified. How are you feeling compared to when we started tapping? Are you still experiencing the upset at the same intensity on the 0 to 10 scale? Has it changed or stayed the same? If nothing has changed, start the exercise again,

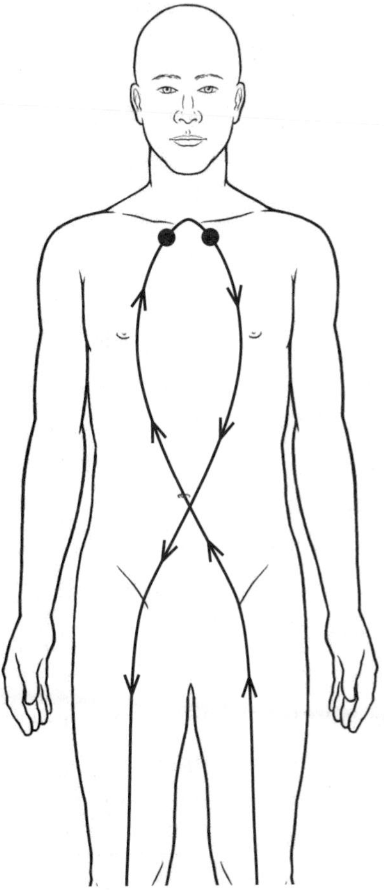

Figure 3: *Tapping on either or both collarbone points activates chi flow in a figure 8 pattern. Just 15 to 30 seconds of tapping or thumping the collarbone points activates chi flow and fosters vitality and wellbeing.*

staying focused on one specific feeling, thought, sensation, or detail of the memory or target you chose. If the intensity has gone up, keep on tapping; you're onto something important! If your intensity has gone down, how far down? You can tap again, just like this, until the upset goes down to 0.

Guessing an Intensity Rating When You're Not Sure

In the beginning, you might not be certain of the intensity of your feeling or upset on the 0 to 10 ratings scale. Don't let a little uncertainty get in the way of your healing—guessing works just fine here.

More on One-Point Tapping: Collarbone Points

Tapping collarbone points benefits your entire body-mind system. According to Traditional Chinese Medicine (TCM) they are master points for rebalancing the body's energy, commonly called the Happiness Points. Chi travels along the meridians in a figure-eight pattern in the body, entering at the left foot, crossing at the navel, and rising near the body's surface at the Chinese acupuncture equivalent of EFT's right collarbone point (the Happiness Point) then to the other collarbone point, and returning to the navel before exiting through the right foot.

On waking in the morning, do one-point tapping for one to five minutes into your morning routine to increase emotional well-being and physical vitality. Tap during your day when you have difficult experiences, uncomfortable thoughts, unpleasant memories, or difficult situations in mind. Tap on that one point continuously for a couple of minutes to shift your mood, thoughts, or painful sensations. If you're at the office or in public, just massage the area gently while focused on the issue. You can also add reassuring phrases or words while tapping, such as "healing this now," or "this problem or feeling is not bigger than I am." You can also tap on this one point as you read.

When you don't have time to perform the full EFT process, one-point tapping works great. Duck into a restroom, pull the car over, or step into an empty hallway to tap. Tapping for just five minutes on the collarbone points moves excess lymph through your body, boosts your immune function, balances your adrenal glands, and gives an overall sense of well-being. What's not to love?

In Conclusion

In this chapter, we've explored what EFT does, a brief history of how EFT developed, and how to do easy, one-point tapping. Next, we jump into hands-on tapping. You'll know how to do the basics of the EFT process by the end of chapter 2.

Chapter 2
How to Tap, Step by Step

Getting Started Hands On with the EFT Basic Recipe

The EFT basic recipe is Gold Standard EFT, the original how-to-tap process, and it's the heart of your EFT toolbox. Use it as a first-aid kit for the bumps and bruises part and parcel of a well-lived life—an antidote for everything from day-to-day distresses to major life upsets. The EFT basic recipe has two distinct parts for each round or cycle of tapping: the EFT setup statement and the EFT sequence.

1. The EFT setup statement: Identify a problem and how intensely you feel about it. Put the problem into the EFT setup formula, and then express it aloud while tapping on the first tapping point known as the Karate Chop point.
2. The EFT sequence: Tap on each of the eight remaining tapping points of the basic recipe while saying a few words that keep you focused on the problem. You can perform this part as many times as you wish—generally until you experience a downward shift in intensity. Together, these two parts are considered one round of tapping.

The EFT basic recipe homes in on the specific target you have chosen to tap on. The continuous tapping stimulates the energy points, essentially dissolving (or neutralizing) the disruption and restoring the energy system's balance. In plain English, you don't feel the upset anymore!

EFT Basic Recipe, Part I

Step 1. Identify a specific problem. In this book, phrases for "the problem" include issue, upset, challenge, distress, tapping opportunity, and tapping target. Tapping targets are usually things you don't like about yourself or a situation, or about something that happened. They are generally things you want to get rid of or wish hadn't happened. They can include feelings, thoughts, beliefs, and body sensations that don't feel good.

Be as specific and clear as possible when you select a target problem. To get long-term results, you need to be specific. Statements such as "my anxiety" or "my stress" are general problem areas. Tapping on the big anxiety you have had for decades will likely provide temporary relief—like a bandage—but it won't get you to the roots of your concern. Getting to the source requires getting into the specific details of your anxiety. You'll learn how to be more specific in chapter 3.

For now, choose a tapping target such as a thought, feeling, experience, or bad memory that brings mild distress or body pain. Here are some mildly distressing examples:

I don't like what my boss just said—it's sexist.
There's no more chicken salad left.
I have this pain in my neck.
I think of that email and get upset.
My toddler is insisting on dressing himself today.
My mosquito bite won't stop itching.

Before moving on to step 2, do another Tarzan tap for 60 seconds. Find the collarbone points, and while tapping repeat any of the positive phrases you said aloud earlier when you one-point tapped. Go ahead and do it now.

Step 2. Determine how much the problem is bothering you on a scale of 0 to 10. The intensity scale is a critical component of EFT; it's your feedback loop. It helps you identify where you are at with an issue, and then it helps you track your progress. Check your intensity after you have done a full tapping round, which you'll do soon. It will help you uncover work still left to do so you can find complete relief. If numbers don't work for you, scale the intensity with your arms: Arms spread wide would be a ten, while palms together would be a zero. Or you can scale the intensity geographically: as small as your house or as big as the world. Find what works for you. If you're unsure, simple guess your level of intensity. Don't think too hard about this. You'll get comfortable with practice.

Step 3. Craft your EFT setup statement. Your setup statement will have two parts:

1. Your problem—that is, the negative tapping target—you phrase like this: "Even though I have (state your problem)...."
2. Your affirmation, something positive about yourself. The standard EFT affirmation is "...I deeply and completely accept myself."

Basic Gold Standard uses the phrase "deeply and completely love and accept myself." Before proceeding, practice deeply and completely accepting yourself right now. Simply insert your target problem into the EFT setup format like so:

> Even though I (have this problem), I deeply and completely accept myself.

The EFT format does not change; it's a negative linked to a positive, but the content—your target problems—will. You can play an infinite number of melodies on the same instrument. For example,

"I don't like what my boss said to me this morning" would look like this: "Even though I don't like what my boss said to me this morning, I deeply and completely accept myself."

Now you have the first part of the EFT basic recipe: the EFT setup statement, which we'll put together with the starting Karate Chop point.

Step 4. Find the location of the Karate Chop point you'll use in the setup.

These instructions describe the use of the left Karate Chop point for clarity. However, you can tap either the left or right Karate Chop point; it all works. Find the Karate Chop point by opening your left hand, pinky side facing down. Using the finger tips or palm of your right hand, tap gently all along the edge of your left palm. This point is named for the hand position karate masters use when they "chop." You can switch hands at any time, if your tapping hand or fingers tire.

Step 5. Repeat the EFT setup statement while tapping the Karate Chop point.

Repeat your EFT setup statement while tapping gently and continuously on the Karate Chop point. This setup aims a spotlight straight at the problem that you have identified as your first tapping target. This alerts the entire central nervous system that you're ready to work. It begins activating and rebalancing your energy system. Combining a negative expression with a positive one neutralizes any subconscious resistance you may have to achieving your goal.

Express your EFT setup statement aloud one or more times while karate chopping. You may have seen it done three times, but Gold Standard has evolved and one time is enough. Gold Standard EFT says once, while others repeat three times. It's really up to you; you won't go wrong repeating your setup statement. You can say the EFT setup silently in your head, shout it out loud, whisper it, whine your way through it, or sing it. The key is to help the upset around your tapping target bubble to the surface.

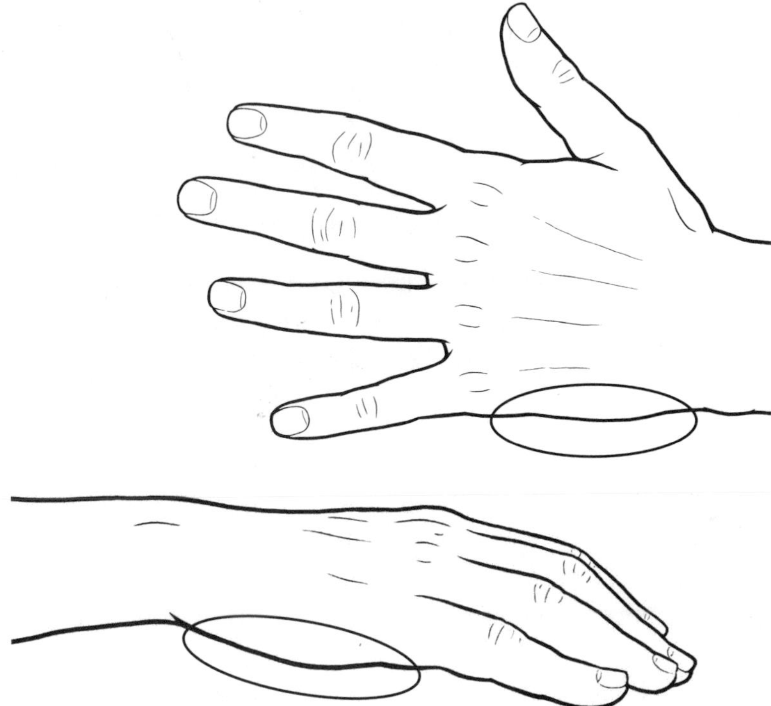

Figure 4: *Karate Chop point, EFT basic recipe starting point. Start the process by karate chopping continuously while expressing your EFT setup statement. The Karate Chop point on the side of the hand corresponds to the small intestine acupuncture meridian. Either hand can be used to chop. Tapping is all along the side of the palm, not just on one point.*

Alternate Starting Point for the Setup: The Sore Spot (SS)

An alternate, equally effective but less common starting point for tapping is the Sore Spot (SS). Find it by "walking" your fingers out from the center of your collarbone, either three inches to the right or left, toward your shoulders. Rub or massage this area gently in a circular motion. The spot is often tender, which is why it's called the Sore Spot (SS).

As with the collarbone points, there are two sore spots, one on each side of the chest. The Sore Spot is *not* the collarbone point. See Figure 5 for clarity and location of the two different tapping areas.

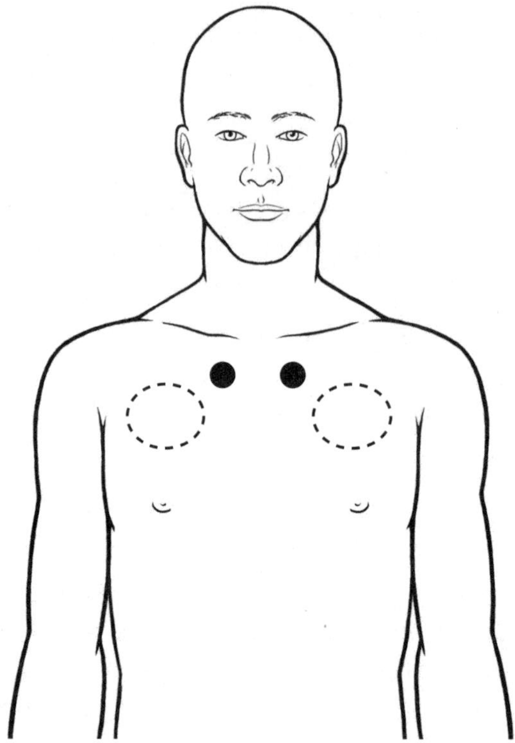

Figure 5: The Sore Spot, an alternate, less used point, can be used instead of the Karate Chop to start the EFT basic recipe and activate the body's energy system.

Step 6. Practice the EFT setup now. Repeat the following EFT setup several times while tapping continuously on your Karate Chop Point or Sore Spot:

> Even though I have this problem, I deeply and completely accept myself.

EFT basic recipe, Part II (The EFT Sequence Reminder Phrase and Eight Energy Points)

You've set up the problem by saying "Even though I have this problem, I deeply and completely accept myself." Now, work on the second part of the EFT basic recipe, the EFT sequence. Tap down the sequence points while expressing a reminder or problem phrase that reminds you of your tapping target.

Step 1: Create an EFT Sequence Reminder Phrase. Sometimes EFT can work so quickly that people forget what they were tapping on. The reminder phrase keeps the spotlight where it belongs, on the targeted problem.

To create a reminder phrase, choose a phrase from your setup statement that elicits the most emotional intensity. Suppose you're upset about what David said on the phone last night. Here's the EFT setup: "Even though I have this upset over what David said on the phone last night, I deeply and completely accept myself." Choose a reminder or problem phrase such as: "upset at what David said," or "my David phone upset," or simply "David upset."

Suppose your EFT setup looks like this: "Even though I am sad about the loss of my dog Cedar who died last month, I deeply and completely accept myself." A reminder phrase might be: "my sadness about Cedar dying," or "Cedar died and I'm sad," or "my Cedar loss." You can even just use the generic "this problem," as your reminder phrase.

If you're upset but can't quite identify what you're feeling, just tune into the feeling happening *right now.* The words are not as critical to success as the feelings—both emotional and physical sensations—relating to the problem. Staying tuned in to the feelings you're experiencing when you focus on the problem is at the heart of EFT. The feelings lead you to resolution, and it's feelings, not words, that become stuck inside your primitive brain. Even if you don't have the right words or are unclear how to say it, EFT will still work if you are tuned in to the upset feeling.

Step 2: Combine reminder phrase with the eight energy points. Repeat the reminder phrase while tapping on the eight tapping points of the EFT tapping sequence, on the head and upper torso (see Figure 6.) Using the index and middle fingers of the left or right hand, tap gently about five to seven times on each point.

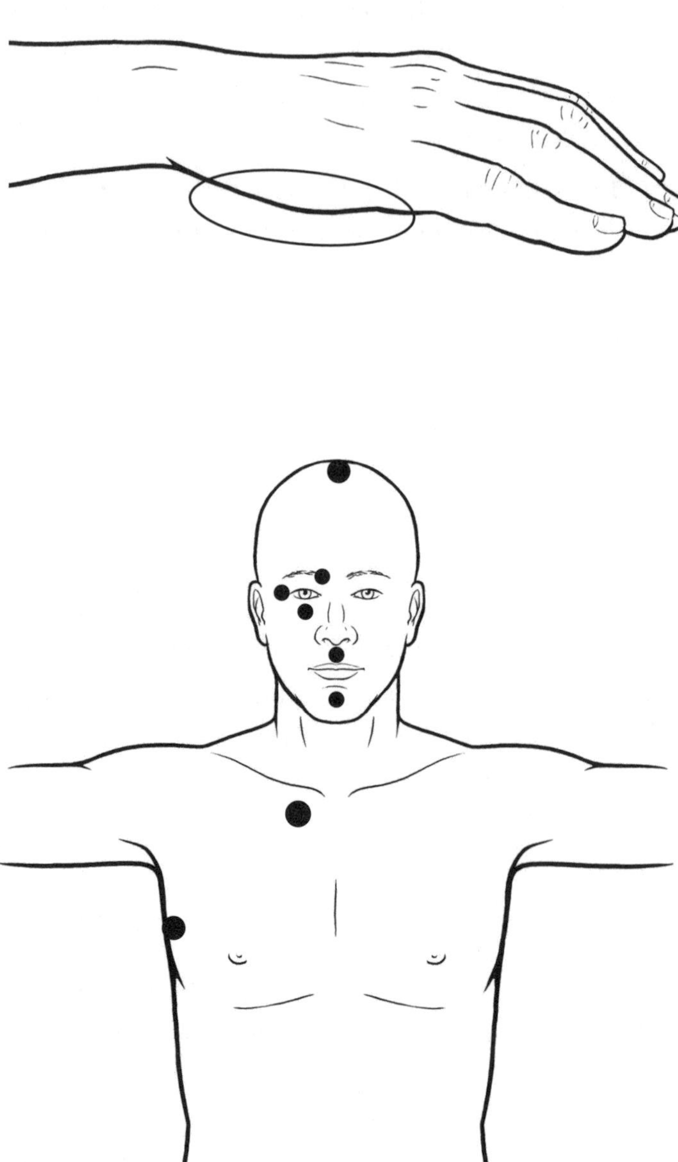

Figure 6: *After the EFT setup statement, where you state your problem while karate chopping, you then apply the EFT Sequence, tapping on the eight points in the order given in the text holding a feeling, body sensation, thought, or image associated with the targeted problem in mind.*

The sequence starts at the top of the head and moves down from there through to your under arm point. Tap on each point five to seven times, with index and middle fingers of either hand. Locate the following tapping sequence points:

Top of Head: Gently tap with palm open wide atop the center or crown of your head for a few seconds or the equivalent of five to seven taps.

Inside of eyebrow: Touch the bridge of your nose, and then move your tapping fingers slightly to the left or to the right to just inside the eyebrow. Tap lightly.

Side of eye: Touch the bony part outside of your eye, and tap lightly; it's about a half-inch from the outside edge of your eye, but not as far as the soft temple spot.

Under eye: Find the bone underneath your eye, under the iris. Tap gently on this under-eye bone, as it may be tender.

Under nose: Tap under your nose in the crease between the nose and upper lip.

Chin: Tap under your lower lip in the indention between your lower lip and chin.

Collarbone: You already know the collarbone point as the Tarzan tapping point.

Under arm: Find this point about four fingers down from the armpit, on the upper rib cage. For women, this would be about at the bra line. When you massage this point a bit deeper, it is often sore. Access these points easily by reaching one arm (e.g., the right) across the body to tap on the other side (e.g., under the left arm). You can tap this point with all four fingers or the flat of your hand and fingers.

When you are tapping, you can switch hands, tap with one or both hands at the same time, tap with all your fingers or just one finger, or cross your hands and tap on opposite sides of your body.

No matter which side you tap, you've stimulated the meridians and activated your body's energy system.

Step 3. Test your intensity after each tapping round. After you tap one full EFT tapping round, return to the original upset you were tapping on and check your intensity level again on the 0 to 10 scale to see what has changed and what's left to work on. Do more rounds if your intensity is higher than 2 before moving on to tap on a different issue.

Now all the pieces of the EFT basic recipe are in place. Let's review:

1. Identify a problem—a troubling feeling, sensation, thought, or bad memory.
2. Rate the current intensity of the problem on the 0 to 10 scale.
3. Insert the problem into the EFT template to create the EFT setup statement.
4. Repeat the EFT setup statement one or more times while continuously tapping the Karate Chop point.
5. Create an EFT reminder phrase that is shorthand for the problem.
6. Tap the eight points of the EFT tapping sequence while repeating the reminder phrase.
7. Test the intensity number again after tapping one or two sequence rounds.
8. Adjust for changes in intensity by tweaking your setup phrase or creating a different setup phrase, and start the process all over again.

This EFT basic recipe summary is also in appendix A along with images of the tapping points for easy access as you move through the rest of the book. If you are not new to tapping, you likely have seen people tapping other points. You may know that the original basic recipe was longer and that it keeps evolving. We'll explore the original basic recipe points toward the chapter's end, as well as other effective tapping points. With more than four-hundred meridian points on our bodies that are all connected, variation is definitely okay.

Exercise: Putting It All Together

Let's practice the whole EFT basic recipe—the EFT setup statement and the EFT sequence—without any specific content. Tap your Karate Chop point while repeating your EFT setup phrase one to three times. In this case, since you are learning, I'll repeat the setup three times:

> ***Karate chop:*** *Even though I have "this problem," I deeply and completely accept myself.*
>
> ***Karate chop:*** *Even though I have "this problem," I deeply and completely accept myself.*
>
> ***Karate chop:*** *Even though I have "this problem," I deeply and completely accept myself.*

Next, follow the setup with the EFT tapping sequence, tapping the points below while saying aloud your reminder or problem phrase about the problem you've targeted.

1. ***Top of head:*** Your reminder/problem phrase.
2. ***Inside eyebrow:*** Your reminder phrase.
3. ***Side of eye:*** Your reminder phrase.
4. ***Under eye:*** Your reminder phrase.
5. ***Under nose:*** Your reminder phrase.
6. ***Chin:*** Your reminder phrase.
7. ***Collarbone:*** Your reminder phrase.
8. ***Under arm:*** Your reminder phrase.

Excellent! You have just completed one round of Gold Standard EFT tapping. People regularly tap through the sequence one or more times, but it still counts as one round until the EFT setup statement changes. See EFT Resources to access video and more written tutorials on the basic recipe.

Exercise: Tapping on a Real Target

Step 1. Identify a mini problem. Since you're just starting out, don't take on your deepest, darkest issues and fears yet. You're in a learning phase. Ask yourself: Is there something that happened earlier today or this week that was mildly upsetting to me? Am I feeling a negative emotion about somebody or something that happened recently? Am I feeling a body ache or pain? As an example, I'll use Matt, who is experiencing tightness around the left shoulder blade from sitting hunched over his computer. Tap along with Matt's problem example below or create your own EFT setup phrase.

Step 2. Rate your current intensity (how you feel right now) about the targeted problem on the 0 to 10 scale, and write that down. Matt's shoulder blade tightness is a 5 on the scale.

Step 3. Create your EFT setup statement to accurately describe the problem. Matt says, "Even though I have this computer tightness feeling in my left shoulder, I deeply and completely accept myself."

Step 4. Repeat the words aloud while tapping continuously on your Karate Chop point. (Remember, you can use your own phrase, or the one provided here.) Matt's statement: "Even though I have this computer tightness feeling in my left shoulder, I deeply and completely accept myself."

Step 5. Tap through the EFT sequence, tapping down the points while expressing the reminder or problem phrase aloud. Matt's reminder phrase might be: "this tightness in my left shoulder due to being hunched over the computer," which is a bit wordy. Saying "tightness in my left shoulder" also reminds him of the problem and keeps his mind, body, and energy system focused there:

Top of head: *Tightness in my left shoulder.*

Inside eyebrow: *Tightness in my left shoulder.*

Side of eye: *Tightness in my left shoulder.*

Under eye: *Tightness in my left shoulder.*

Under nose: *Tightness in my left shoulder.*

Chin: *Tightness in my left shoulder.*

Collarbone: *Tightness in my left shoulder.*

Under arm: *Tightness in my left shoulder.*

You'll notice that all the words were the same in this tapping sequence. This makes it much easier to focus on the precise detail that you are tapping on and to make sure your body-mind is tuned into the problem. To avoid confusion as you begin your learning and to lay a solid foundation for more advanced EFT later, we'll apply the same reminder phrase wording used in the earlier stages. As you learn more, you can use phrases that are within the scope of your EFT setup statement, such as: "It really hurts," "it's so tight," "ouch it hurts," "this tight left shoulder," "this tight shoulder feeling on my left side."

Step 6. Get feedback by testing your results. Matt started out with a 5 in intensity on his left shoulder tightness on the 0 to 10 scale. Now the tightness level has subsided to a 2.

....

After each tapping round, remember to ask yourself: Am I still feeling the same, or has the intensity gone up or down? Write your number on the intensity scale and compare it with the intensity with which you began. Writing it out helps you recognize any shifts you have made and guides you to where you should go in your next tapping round. What if you notice that another detail or aspect of this problem is now bothering you? This simply means you have tapped down the first aspect enough to allow the next aspect or detail in line to rise to the surface, and that's progress. Ideally you tap your first target down to a 0 or at least below a 2 before moving on, or you'll have blowback.

Understanding the concept of aspects (components or details) of a problem is important for understanding the feedback you receive from the 0 to 10 scale and for effectively targeting your ongoing EFT work on yourself.

What to Do When Intensity Subsides, Increases, or Stays the Same

When you start out as a tapper, it can be challenging to specifically separate out every detail of a problem, rate your feelings, or even know *what* you are feeling. Your skills will improve as you learn to think in terms of aspects and intensity. For now, if you are finding this too difficult, go ahead and do a minute of one-point tapping and then continue on. Or perform the EFT basic recipe, naming your intensity on the 0 to 10 scale, using this EFT setup phrase: "Even though this is too hard, I deeply and completely accept myself." Reminder phrase: "this is too hard." Retest your intensity when you are done.

After One Round—Intensity lower: If your intensity on the 0 to 10 scale has dropped, it means that you are experiencing some relief from the problem. A rating of 0 means that the issue no longer bothers you. If you have a little remaining intensity, you can tap about any other detail that is troubling you that's related to the original problem. In Matt's case, it would be anything else that is bothering him or that comes to mind as he tapped or as he thinks about the tightness in his shoulder. You can use this new information to adjust your original setup phrase to reflect the changes you experience or to develop a new setup phrase. If the intensity is low enough, move on to the next issue.

Intensity higher: If your intensity has gone higher, keep tapping! This means that you're tuned in to the target and that there's a lot of intensity you've been sitting on. The good news? The feelings and sensations around the issue are releasing as you tap. Keep going until you feel complete relief. The tapping is literally forcing the disruption to resolve itself. Emotional gushers are a good sign of release and relief, in most cases. However, in some situations, when there is undiagnosed or unresolved significant trauma, if the intensity remains high and you experience ongoing upset over hours or days, seek resources outside of yourself, including a mental health professional and an ACEP-accredited EFT professional.

Intensity same: No change could mean a couple of things. The EFT setup statement may be too general. If Matt's "tight left shoulder" has the same intensity as when he started tapping, he might require a sharper focus to get results, such as: "this tight, sharp point about the size of a pencil point just inside my left shoulder blade."

No change could also mean you're sitting on an emotional present that perhaps has more than a few layers of gift-wrap around it. Be persistent. Maybe part of the problem you are tapping on is not as big a deal as another detail or aspect of the problem. For example, if you are tapping for the problem of: "my difficulty meeting a decent man/woman," and the intensity of 7 is not budging, you might look for issues that might be getting in the way of experiencing relief. These could be: "my anger at my ex," which is a 10, and "my sadness that I'm alone again," which is also a 10. The emotions underlying these issues may be at the core of the energy disruption. You may need to address them first before the difficulty can be resolved.

Sometimes shifting aspects may be behind apparent lack of headway on a problem. This means that while you tap on one specific issue, such as "sadness about the loss," you're feeling many things: anger, sadness, frustration, upset, annoyance, self-pity, and more. The issue might not be shifting because you're feeling all these things at once. In time, you must tease these various aspects out and tap on them one at a time to get results. At first, they may be all jumbled together like a big knotted ball of yarn.

As detailed at this chapter's end, tapping additional points is helpful when you're stuck. I have found them effective when I'm having a hard time moving down the intensity scale and when the intensity is quite high, as well. Sometimes the issue can be better handled with the help of a supportive person working with you to get the results you know you can achieve, including a therapist or a seasoned and proven EFT practitioner. Be prepared to make that call when you need it.

The EFT Spiral: When Aspects Lead to Core Issues

It is typically the case in my own practice that the problem of the day, even if minor, pings off earlier traumatic events, often early childhood traumas. Even if no logical link exists between the "today" upset and the past, that's okay, we're working with the subconscious which has a "mind" all its own. Ask yourself "what does this problem remind me of? Have I ever experienced something like this before?" Then go to that "before" problem and tap on that. The earlier you go, the more likely you will address the cause that set in motion patterns that have troubled you for years.

When you aim EFT at the earlier experience, you have the opportunity to resolve not just the minor current problem, but also the root cause from back in the day. Once these historic emotional traumas release, you might feel like your whole world has changed. EFT is not a linear process. It's more like a spiral process.

So when you tap about a teeny, weeny, seemingly superficial upset on the outside of that spiral, you may also be working through a deeper issue at the heart of that same spiral, and vice versa. When you're working on one event, you are in a sense working on all events housed in that same energy disruption. Assume in most cases that even when you are jumping in with the small stuff, you are working on a number of levels at the same time. In the long run, when you grow more comfortable with EFT, you'll start at any point on the spiral—from the deep, dark interiors all the way to the little wiggly tail.

With Matt's troublesome shoulder, here are some aspects or details that he did tap on: "This is where I injured my shoulder before; I'm scared it's going to get worse; why did I help my sister move that piano yesterday?!" Each of these would be a separate round of tapping. Lest you think this will take too many minutes from your life, ask yourself how much the problem is costing you now. Then time one tapping round. It takes all of 30 to 60 seconds.

Matt addresses these aspects and now feels almost no shoulder pain at all. Is he done? If there is more work to be done, something else may come to mind, such as a bothersome thought, image, past upsetting experience, question, or sudden idea about what the target problem is attached to. The arising of other thoughts and issues is completely normal; consider it a marvelous hallmark of EFT and a taste of what can happen when you harness it for your healing benefit.

As Matt focuses in again on the shoulder, a fleeting thought comes to mind: his big work project deadline. He now realizes he's been holding himself so tight in the shoulder because of the tight project deadline bearing down hard on his shoulders and frustration about his colleague who hasn't been pulling his fair share of the project's weight. This is a different issue from the pain in the shoulder; it's part of what's holding up the pain in the shoulder. Matt crafts a different EFT setup statement to reflect this. In accordance with our EFT spiral, Matt's present issue is stretching back to an earlier or core energy disruption from childhood. There was the time when his father expected him to do something beyond Matt's abilities—he had no idea how to do it. Matt might have felt that performing under this heavy burden was the only way he could get approval or love from his father. Here is the core issue where the energy disruption began.

The outermost symptom on the EFT spiral—the tight shoulder of today—leads Matt to a core unresolved problem from his childhood at the spiral heart: the need to take on heavy burdens without help in order to gain approval. So the tight shoulder might be an opening to address with EFT core unresolved painful experiences and events from his childhood. Eventually his tight left shoulder would be a thing of the past or a welcome reminder that he is taking on too much work or pushing himself too hard while neglecting to acknowledge how well he is doing. Later we'll discuss in more detail how a simple issue can lead to clearing a chain or pattern of negative emotions.

Can you see how EFT could benefit Matt? His physical shoulder pain could disappear completely. He would remember to stretch more often at work and wouldn't snap at coworkers. He could ask for help and address team slacker issues, no longer terrorized by deadline problems. He would feel more energized and vital at home and at work.

Thinking, feeling, and acting differently come with the territory of EFT results. Recall the image of the small stone in the still pond: the ripples radiate from the center and affect the whole body of water. EFT ripples will change your life in surprising ways.

Insights and shifts like Matt's are par for the course, even when you are new to tapping. They are called cognitive shifts in EFT parlance. By its nature, when performed appropriately, EFT goes deep.

Going Deeper: Welcoming the Bad Feelings, Expressing Affirmations, and More

We welcome bad feelings with EFT, but not because we're gluttons for punishment—quite the opposite. The problems are opportunities for us to reconnect with parts of ourselves that were shut down or abandoned in order to cope. Now we receive ourselves back.

Targeting the Negative

Some clients initially resist saying the negatives. With EFT, we say the negative to allow it to clear, not to feed the fire. Focusing on the negative with the EFT setup statement does not mean that you are indulging in your problems or complaining or that you're going to attract even more negativity into your life. You are popping the big fear balloon you've been carrying inside and removing the power it has over you.

By acknowledging the negative problem while tapping, we actually stop pushing it down and start allowing it to flow through and out of our body, mind, and energy system. Intentionally allowing ourselves to feel what we actually feel about a problem releases the troubling emotions around it, and our bodies experience a corresponding relief, as they never lie. Living in present time, our bodies are incapable of lying. Tapping will resolve the energy disruption, bring relief, and allow our system to rebalance.

By pairing the negative with the positive and staying focused on a specific tapping target, we can resolve the problem thought, feeling, belief, or memory with minimal pain and discomfort.

More on Choosing the Tapping Target: Specific Versus Global and Tabletops

First, clearly identify the problem you're experiencing. Then home in on the specific part or aspect of the problem that's most bothersome. Taking on the whole ball of wax is overwhelming, so finding the one thing about the problem that troubles you most provides a simple and achievable task.

Ask yourself thoughtful questions, and give yourself a minute or two to realize what's causing your present upset. Are you feeling tense because of all the traffic? Was it that phone call a moment ago, when the boss took out her anger on you? Are you just feeling tired and out of sorts because you're bored? Do you have a sinus headache or toothache?

Tapping asks us to slow down a moment and check in: "What feels off or really wrong right now?" Then we get to do something about it. If it feels too hard yet to identify a target, one way to ease yourself into tapping is simply to tap and talk about the issue bothering you. This means you tap while you are talking about something that is upsetting you, which could include a body ache or pain. Tapping while talking will bring you some relief, because it is activating the body's life-energy system and pushing the upset through. You can also tap while you are talking on the phone.

Tabletops and Table Legs: General, Specific, and Global in EFT

Overall issues—depression, grief, a phobia, weight—are general, global, with many different parts, details, and aspects. Think of these larger issues as tabletops held up by many specific table legs, each of which is an event holding up the tabletop, and that's what we want to work with. Tap to zero enough specific events (legs) holding up the big tabletop of anxiety and the whole thing collapses. So no, you don't have to tap on every little thing that's gone wrong in your life…what a relief! That effect is known as the "Generalization Effect" in EFT.

Let's look at a few examples of general versus specific:

GENERAL	SPECIFIC
feelings of worry	worried my child is still not home at midnight
my food issue	can't stop eating potato chips
anxious in school	seeing Steve the bully in gym
boyfriend/girlfriend problems	when he/she said, "It might be over."
bad childhood memories	the night my parent threw me out in the snow

To get specific, get curious. If you're dealing with anxiety ask: "When do I have the anxiety?" "What does this feeling remind me of?" "When was the last time I experienced the anxiety?" "What proof do I have of the anxiety?" "What was happening in my life when my anxiety first started?" "Where do I feel anxiety in my body?" The answers produce specific tapping targets. The "what does this remind me of?" question is one you'll turn to again and again to uncover specific events.

Here's another example for a person upset about "the divorce." Choose specific experiences along the divorce timeline: "finding out about the cheating," "opening the bill from the lawyer," "the hateful way my spouse looked at me across the table at mediation," "telling the kids," etc. Think of these memories as moments in time.

It may take a little practice breaking down problems, events, or feelings, but soon it'll be second nature.

Name Your Targeted Event, Review It as if It Were a Movie

It is also helpful to give the target you are tapping on a name, such as, "worry about my son," or "potato chip fiasco," or "bully fear." Consider it as if you are using your event to title a book or a scene in a movie. Then, once you have tapped the target down to zero, run through the whole thing as if it were a movie, scene by scene, and tap down any remaining intensity including sensations, upsetting details, or images and thoughts. You comb through the scenes of the movie trying to raise intensity, because if you leave any outstanding intensity, the weeds aren't pulled out at the roots and the event will come back to bother you again.

Balancing Negative and Positive

The classic EFT affirmation phrase is, "I deeply and completely accept myself." Not surprisingly, people sometimes feel uncomfortable thinking or saying this, asking, "What if I really don't?" "What if I can't honestly say that?" "Isn't it wrong to accept a certain part of myself that I want to change? Doesn't that mean I'm giving up?"

You don't have to believe the acceptance phrase, but an affirmation is part of the process. If you are having a hard time thinking anything positive about yourself—and this is a common challenge for people new to EFT—what *do* you feel good about? Use that as your affirmation phrase, for example: "I love the park down the street from my house," or "my friend's four-year-old is so completely alive," or "this is a beautiful day," or "I love my kitty cat, Mr. Purr," or "I love to______" (you name it).

More advanced work might have you tapping on all the negative feelings that come up when you say or think about the phrase: "I deeply and completely accept myself." In this case, tap till you feel comfortable saying, "I deeply and completely accept myself."

Incidentally, the resistance that comes up as a result of saying you love and accept yourself is called a tail-ender in EFT. It means that you've flushed out something else to tap on. These are also known as "yes-buts." Tail-enders and yes-buts show you where the resistance is. Just tapping on tail-ender or yes-but resistance can be a richly rewarding experience. Use it for your healing. If you're like most of us, you've already beaten yourself up enough in this lifetime, so be patient with yourself.

Other acceptance phrases that work include:

- I really want to completely accept myself.
- I love, honor, accept, and forgive myself.
- I'm okay.
- Maybe someday I can accept myself.
- I accept myself and how I feel.
- I love, honor, accept, and forgive myself.

Find a place of positive truth that feels just right to you. Accepting yourself even though you have a problem helps the part of you that's stuck realize that you are more than just the problem: you have intrinsic worth no matter how you feel, what you look like, what "bad" things you've done, or what's happened in your life. It's the big picture of you that sees your value and worth all the time, the higher self that sees you as far more than just the upset you are feeling in the moment. Likewise, you need to be in the present to make a change.

Apex Effect: Going Deeper with the Intensity Scale and Aspects

The intensity scale is a critical component of EFT. Don't skip over it! If you do, you might be subject to the apex effect, which is when a person forgets that he or she actually had a problem and doesn't even remember tapping on it. Sometimes it will even happen in the middle of a tapping round; that's how quickly EFT can work.

I once tapped with my friend Scott on his decades-long snuffling and snorting problem from a deviated septum after walking into the side of a barn when he was twenty years old. This problem had plagued him personally and professionally; it made him look socially inept, the sound was off-putting, and it worsened in uncomfortable social situations. We tapped on all aspects relating to this problem, from the social issues to the benefits of not having to socialize because the snort was off-putting, from the sound to the initial trauma, and to the fact that he didn't have to have it because both he and his nose had survived. The snorting disappeared that night and never returned. He forgot he had ever been a "social snorter." All this to illustrate why writing down your setup statement and your intensity rating in your EFT journal is important. You need to track your progress and get feedback, especially when you are feeling low. Seeing in your journal that change is possible and that you have already made phenomenal strides in your healing work is a great boost. It helps restore hope to its rightful place of honor.

Limiting Beliefs: What If I Can't Do this "Right"?

Are you wondering if EFT will really work for you? Are you worried you won't be able to do it right, or do you feel overwhelmed by all the information? Maybe you're afraid of what will happen if you make big changes in your life. If any of this is happening right now, take a look at these setups to see if they resonate with you. We will use the first phrase here as the example:

1. "Even though I don't know if EFT will work for me, I love, honor, and accept myself."
2. Rate your intensity when you express this aloud. How true does this feel to you on the 0 to 10 scale?
3. Express the EFT setup statement: **Karate chop:** "Even though I don't know if EFT will work for me, I love, honor, and accept myself."
4. Tap through the EFT sequence.

    Top of head: I don't know if tapping will work for me.

Inside eyebrow: This might not work for me.
Side of eye: This might not work for me.
Under eye: Afraid tapping won't work for me.
Under nose: I don't know if this will work.
Chin: Afraid this won't work for me.
Collarbone: I don't know if tapping will really work.
Under arm: This might not work for me.

5. Retest your intensity. Do you believe as strongly that it won't work for you?

Other sample phrases to consider tapping one round on:

> Even though I'm not willing to say all that negative stuff about what's going on, I deeply and completely accept myself.
>
> Even though I'm afraid of change, I accept myself anyway.
>
> Even though this feels really hard, I'm open to doing it anyway.
>
> Even though I don't understand how something this easy could possibly help me solve my kind of problems, I deeply and completely accept myself.
>
> Even though I don't think I can get this right, I deeply and completely accept myself.

Tapping on the truth about what you're *really* thinking can be transformative—and come up more quickly than you think. Choose any of these phrases that resonate with you and tap on it. You might find things feel easier, lighter, and more possible after just a few tapping rounds. Try a few rounds now.

Additional Useful Tapping Points: the Nine Gamut, Finger Points, and More

The original EFT basic recipe used to have more points. Other energy-meridian tapping practitioners also use a wide range of tapping points and approaches. The points that were in the original recipe include finger points and the nine gamut points.

The fingertip and gamut series were performed after one full round of the EFT basic recipe. However, as EFT has distilled into Gold Standard EFT, in the majority of cases, neither finger points nor gamut points are essential. Use these points when you're not getting expected results with the EFT basic recipe or when dealing with a stubborn aspect. I apply it with clients and on myself when tsunami-type feelings—sobbing, rage, or acute pain spikes—arise or when feeling stuck. It seems to move the upset through faster. I'll use them maybe once or twice in a sixty-minute tapping session. The gamut process also resonates with people who have experienced the trauma-treatment therapy known as Eye Movement Desensitization and Reprocessing (EMDR), those who know that crossing the midline helps with left-right brain integration and enhances a person's ability to learn, or those who have tried REM (Rapid Eye Movement) therapy. The process accesses both sides of the brain and helps to integrate left and right hemispheres so you access whole-brain thinking.

Take note of all of these point locations, and experiment on your own with them. You will be encouraged to try these points while reading as you continue to test the process. All of these points can be found in appendix A along with images for easy reference as you continue on through the rest of the book.

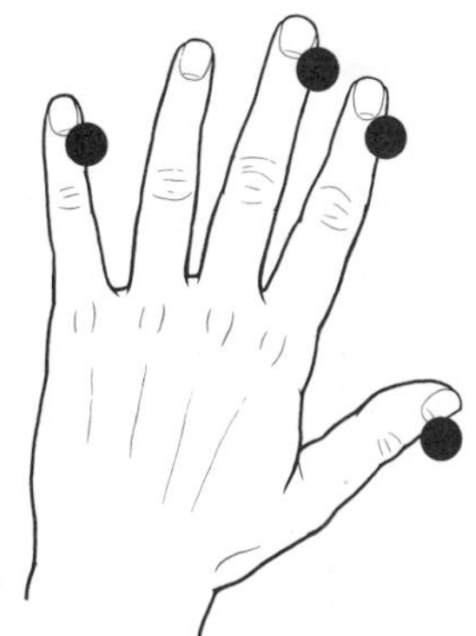

Fingertip Points

After one round EFT tapping round, start tapping on the tip side of the thumb of either hand, the side facing away from the index finger. Then tap on the side tip of the index finger, the side nearest your thumb. Follow through with each finger except the ring finger in the same manner. The ring finger is not tapped because the meridian for this is on the other side of the fingertip. It's faster and easier to stay with the routine of inside finger-point tapping. Some practitioners rely mainly on the finger points as part of their tapping protocol.

The finger points are also useful when you can't tap on all the points because you're in an office meeting or you're in another place where you don't want to appear conspicuous. Just drum with your fingertips on your body or on the tabletop, or just bring your hands together and tap one against the other—no one will know you're tapping. The fingertip points can also be used when you have difficulty reaching the other basic recipe tapping points.

I use the finger points in combination with the nine gamut. First the finger points, then the nine gamut series.

Please note that fingertip points will come in handy as you tap and read throughout the text. I'll also be asking you at regular intervals to tap on these finger points, the collarbone point, or the EFT sequence points, as you'll soon see.

Nine Gamut Series

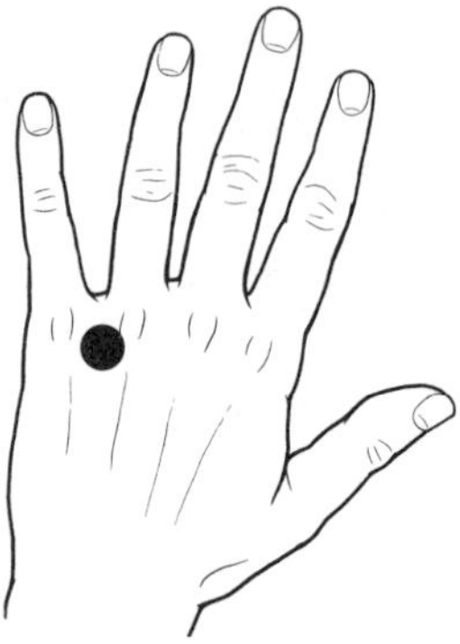

After tapping the fingertip points, tap on the top of either hand, just behind the knuckle and the V formed by the ring finger and the pinkie (the gamut point), while doing nine different things. The left-right action harnesses and integrates both creative and logical sides of your brain.

While tapping on the gamut point on either hand:

1. Close your eyes.
2. Open your eyes, and look up as high as you can without moving your head.
3. Look down to the far right while keeping your head steady and straight ahead.

4. Look down to the far left while keeping your head steady and straight ahead.
5. Fully circle your eyes clockwise starting at 12:00.
6. Fully circle your eyes counterclockwise starting at 12:00.
7. Hum two seconds of a song that has no negative emotional charge associated with it. You want a song that does not stimulate a bad memory. I often use "Twinkle Twinkle Little Star."
8. Count to five.
9. Hum two seconds of song.

Next:

1. Repeat the EFT sequence, tapping down the eight points using the reminder phrase.
2. Then test your results, rating your feeling about the tapping target on the 0 to 10 scale. If you still haven't resolved the issue completely, look for other aspects, and tap on those using the EFT basic recipe.

Below Nipple Points/Liver Points

The "below nipple" points are just under the breast, directly below the nipple, one on each side. They are often omitted because they can be awkward to access, but I like tapping on these because the liver is often associated with anger.

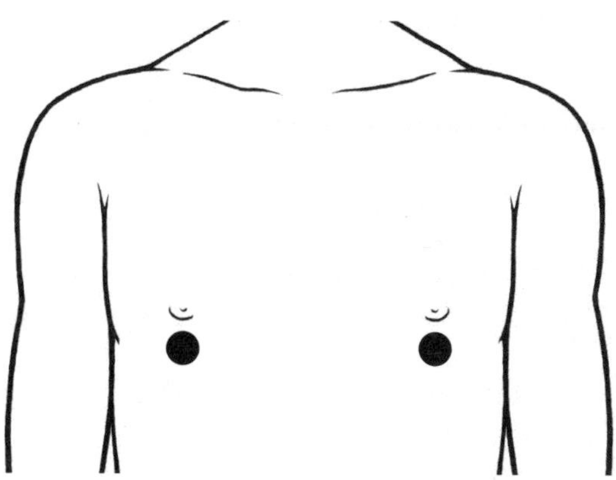

Wrist Points

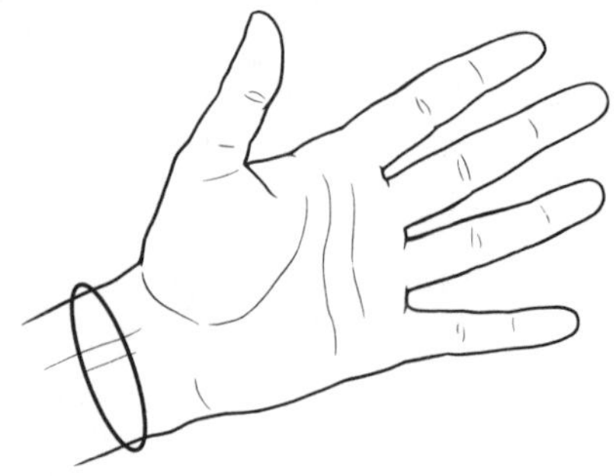

You can tap on the insides of the wrists about three finger-widths down from where your hand starts. You can tap the inside and then the outside of one wrist with the inside of the other or use the fingers of one hand to tap the inside of the other wrist.

To review, although the basic recipe involving the Karate Chop point or Sore Spots and the sequence of eight points are normally all you need, the nine gamut series and the finger, liver, and wrist points can be used in addition when you are not making headway, when there is significant upset, or just to see how things change for you when you try these points.

In Conclusion

Now that you know the basics of how to tap with Gold Standard EFT, why we tap on the negative and positive, what an aspect is, how to check your intensity on the intensity ratings scale, and how to experiment with other tapping points, you're ready for chapter 3. You'll discover how to efficiently identify what to tap on, tools to clear long-standing challenges, and surprising tips and tricks for using EFT on complicated issues. Ready for more?

Chapter 3
Getting Specific, Getting Results

A common mistake people make with EFT is not being specific enough in the stories they are tapping on. They don't get the results they expect and then quit. But really, these people just needed to get more specific about their tapping target.

Getting to the heart of an event is sort of like reading a good book: you need the details to get caught up in the story. The same is true when you are unsticking places in your heart, body, mind, and energy system with EFT tapping. You go into the heart of a troubling memory to release its hold over you, and you do that by uncovering the specific details of the memory, aspect by aspect, tapping on them one at a time all the way down to zero, until you experience neutrality and relief when you think about that targeted memory again.

In the first part of this chapter, we'll explore different ways we can get specific to get results:

1. Differentiating between the global or the big, overall tabletop issues, as opposed to specific events or table legs.
2. Creating specific EFT setup statements;
3. Uncovering and tapping on aspects, or the unique details or components of a specific event; and

4. Working with the individual, separate events that make up a global issue.

When I first started tapping on my own, the effect was fast, easy, and encouraging. I figured I'd resolve everything: the fibromyalgia, self-sabotage, single-mama resentments, longstanding simmering anger at my ex, and of course all the humiliations from childhood and bad memories in just a few tapping rounds. It was, er, slightly overly optimistic!

Tapping on, say, the big issue of my fibromyalgia (I said, "Even though I have fibromyalgia, I deeply and completely accept myself"), my self-sabotage ("Even though I sabotage myself, I deeply and completely accept myself"), my childhood humiliations, and the like didn't get me very far on the road to relief. In fact, these issues were too general—they were the tabletop, global concerns held up by troubling specific table leg events from the past. To get a handle on the global issues, I had to get specific. I got curious about my issues and started asking myself a lot of open-ended questions.

Taking my self-sabotage as an example, I came to wonder along these lines: *When did I sabotage? In what areas of my life did I sabotage? Was there a pattern to my self-sabotage? What was happening in my life right before I began one of the sabotage cycles? What are the pegs or memories holding up my self-sabotage? When was the first time I ever sabotaged that I can remember? What negative talk, big feelings, and beliefs come to mind when I did sabotage or when I was stepping out of my comfort zone and hadn't yet sabotaged?*

These questions gave me a plethora of specific events to tap on. These events (tapping targets) were legs holding up the global issue, self-sabotage. After resolving the emotional intensity on many specific tapping targets, including tapping on the details in each event that had intensity for me and vividly visualizing the upsets to uncover any unresolved aspects, I began to make great strides in all areas of my life. And while EFT wasn't the only healing work I did, it was one of the main catalysts in my transformation. It gave me a way to access the emotional drivers holding certain problems in place.

As we continue, go ahead and tap continuously on the fingertip points (see appendix A for an illustration) or practice tapping on the EFT sequence points continuously. While not Gold Standard EFT, tapping continuously will help you absorb the material faster.

Global Issues versus Specific Events

Global tapping on an issue such as "my anxiety" as the feelings arise will likely give you some surface relief, but it won't get you to the cause or roots of your anxiety. Tapping on even one specific anxious event, as it is called in EFT, is going to pay off in the long run and in most cases build the foundation for clearing your anxiety at its roots.

Your anxious event could be when you saw that an email blaming you for a work problem had been copied to your boss and your colleagues; you felt the whole world closing in on you. It could be that time long ago on the first day of kindergarten when you didn't want to let go of your mom's hand and walk through the big doors alone, terrified of being lost for good. It could be when you were eight and felt anxious watching Mom and Dad argue in the kitchen that one night, feeling like your whole world was ending. It could be your anxious feeling when anticipating the SAT coming up on Monday as the test-taker or the parent of the test-taker.

Each of these "anxious" events an be tapped individually. Tapping into the feelings, sensations, thoughts, and beliefs that accompany anxious events accesses and resolves the energy disruption, causing you to experience freedom from anxiety as a result.

There may be a few or dozens or hundreds of specific events under global issues. Clear or neutralize enough of them—three, twenty, or a hundred—and your global problem collapses all the way to its roots, thanks to the Generalization Effect. EFT's effects will ripple out so you don't have to tap on every little upsetting event in your life. Whew!

This works because similar anxious events are filed under the same folder named "Anxiety," if you will. By tapping on one, the subconscious is also working on unraveling others in that file. When situations that once caused anxiety are revisited, there is now neutrality where you once felt upset and angst. You may feel anxious again, but not at the same high level, which just means you have uncovered another aspect.

Start with a Specific Event

You can start with any specific memory that has intensity for you. The earliest childhood memories can have more impact in collapsing the global issue because they're more foundational and may have laid the groundwork for later, similar events you have experienced. But you don't need to go right there just yet—you're learning. For now, just remember that these early events are considered core issues.

In my practice, when a client presents with a "today" problem, I will ask about the first time they felt that problem feeling. Often there will be a first time and a specific memory related to it. Another question that helps uncover specific events include: What's the one thing that happened to you that you wish you could have skipped?

"What does this feeling or event remind me of?" is important to ask yourself—it may bring you right back to a core memory. Here's an example of what I mean. Let's say that John fell and hurt his right shoulder. The shoulder should have recovered by now but it isn't getting better. When we tap on the shoulder pain, what emerges is memories of growing up as the oldest of twelve kids and having to "shoulder" the brunt of family responsibility when he was little because his parents were overwhelmed. They leaned on him hard to help out. The pain of today is sitting atop the unresolved heavy burdens he carried as a youngster. Now he has the opportunity to clear the early events and when he does, the shoulder pain resolves of its own accord.

What if you can't isolate a specific event or time under your global or tabletop issue? Again, looking at the issue of anxiety, maybe it seems like you experience anxiety all the time. Start where you are. Go ahead with a global round of tapping on your feelings of anxiety. Your EFT setup statement would look like this: "Even though I have this anxiety, I deeply and completely accept myself." Something more specific relating to your anxiety will often come to mind.

For example, my client Shirley said she couldn't remember a time when she *didn't* feel anxious; she couldn't isolate a specific anxious event. After one global tapping round, I again asked her what the earliest time she remembered feeling anxious was. A forgotten memory bubbled up from her subconscious without her even having to think about it: "I was four or five and hiding from Mom because she was trying to spank me." Shirley had both a physical sensation as she thought of the memory as well as some emotional intensity. I asked her: "If this was a scene in a movie, what would this scene's title be?" Giving the event you are about to tap on a title helps provide a bit of emotional distance, and it also gives you an easily made reminder phrase. She named the specific tapping target "Hiding from Mom," and that's where we started our work. After tapping through just this one specific event, she found herself feeling much more resilient when faced with situations in which anxiety would normally occur. Incidentally, as you start asking questions in this way, you will find it common for long-submerged memories to bubble up.

Shirley's "Hiding from Mom" memory had all the hallmarks we needed for a tapping target:

1. It was a specific event.
2. It had intensity.
3. It had a beginning, middle, and end.
4. It was under three minutes in length in real time.
5. There was one big emotional crescendo and several smaller emotional spikes of feelings as she recalled the event right now in present-day time.

Now we'll begin to explore how to move from a general complaint to a more specific event and why that's important. Let's look a little closer at how to get specific in an EFT setup statement.

Getting Specific with Your EFT Setup Statement

The following examples will help you understand the difference between a general and a specific "tappable." Compare the general and specific phrases below that cover the same issue. Which phrase is more interesting, drawing you deeper into the story?

Situation 1: A person with low self-esteem

Global: "Even though I have low self-esteem, I deeply and completely accept myself."

Specific: "Even though my feeling that I'm not as good as everyone else hurts my career, I deeply and completely accept myself."

More Specific: "Even though I totally clammed up at the staff meeting when they asked me a question because I was afraid they'd see how dumb I am, I deeply and completely accept myself."

Situation 2: A person depressed about his divorce

Global: "Even though I feel sad about my divorce, I deeply and completely accept myself."

Specific: "Even though I'm sad not living at home since the divorce, I deeply and completely accept myself."

More Specific: "Even though watching the kids walk in the door last night after I dropped them off at what used to be our house, I deeply and completely accept myself."

Situation 3: A person with chronic pain

Global: "Even though I hurt all over my body, I deeply and completely accept myself."

Specific: "Even though the pain on my right side is burning and throbbing, I deeply and completely accept myself."

More Specific: "Even though the pain on the right side of my back feels like a sharp, red-hot needle stabbing me, I deeply and completely accept myself."

Which of the EFT setups place you directly in the situation so you can really feel and see it clearly? Which ones do you think will more effectively help you find the source of the problem and get relief? Exactly.

Not all of the previous examples conform to the structure of beginning-middle-end and two minutes or less as described above. For example, "looking right now at those four stacks of papers piled so high on my dining room table is totally overwhelming" is ongoing every time that person looks at the papers; "the pain on the right side of my back feels like a sharp, red-hot needle stabbing me" is an ongoing concern. That's okay. Thankfully, there are exceptions to every rule in life. I am offering you general guidelines to navigate your way through this work. Trust your judgment and you'll do fine. And please note, this way of chunking down problems takes time—no one expects you to get it right away. Tap, tap, tap…if you're a perfectionist who needs to get things right!

Exercise: Creating Specific EFT Setup Statements

Take out your EFT journal or open your EFT file. We'll target three general or global issues you want to address. You might title this section "Global Versus Specific EFT Setups." We are now going to create three global EFT setups and then see how to get specific with each one of them.

As you start working on this exercise, consider tapping as you read. Doing so will help ease any intensity that arises as you begin delving into areas of your life that bring discomfort. Consider the

Tarzan tap, the finger points, or the tap-down points from the EFT sequence while reading. See chapter 2 for illustrations if you need a refresher.

Step 1. List one or more global problems in your life you'd like to see change or you'd like to feel better about, areas in which you've struggled. Examples include: my overeating, my anxiety, my "mom" stuff, I'm a horrible parent, my feeling of hopelessness, my consistent relationship sabotage, my performance anxiety, my low self-esteem, my chronic pain, my grief, or my feeling of being overwhelmed.

Create an EFT setup, one at a time. "Even though I have this (insert your problem), I deeply and completely accept myself."

Step 2. Now answer one or more of these questions about each global tapping target. Remember, even one question and answer will do as a good start. You can only work with one thing at a time. Examples: How do I know I have this problem? What does this "today" problem remind me of from the past? What situations bring this problem up for me? What else happens when I am having this problem? Can I name these situations as if they were scenes in a movie and list them one at a time? When does this problem happen most often? Who am I around when this happens? How long have I had this problem? What happens inside my body when I experience this problem? What thoughts and beliefs do I have when I think about this problem? What other events does this problem remind me of? What is happening around me or just before I start having this problem? When was the earliest time I can remember having this problem?

Step 3. Now that you have a good amount of information about your global topic, see how many specific events you can find relating to the global topic. Ask yourself if your tapping target has a beginning, middle, and end. Is it two minutes or less in length? Give a short title to each of your tapping targets. Is there at least one emotional spike you feel when you think of the tapping target?

Step 4. List as many tapping targets as you wish under each of your global setup statements. Remember, you will be working on them one at a time. Now that you have a pile of specific events, do you see how you can create much more specific EFT setup statements? These will be far more sharp-edged than the global EFT setups or setups you already created in Step 1. Asking curious questions can help you travel into the specific events and stories holding a global problem in place. Keep these handy: you can use them as tapping examples throughout the book as well as for your own tapping later on.

Getting Even More Specific with Aspects

We just covered global problems versus specific tapping targets. With Gold Standard EFT, we also emphasize getting specific within each tapping target.[7] Each tapping target can have multiple components or details that are upsetting. These components are called "aspects," briefly introduced in chapter 2. Whether you tap on an upsetting event that happened, a performance issue, or a physical issue, there will be aspects of intensity. Clear the aspects and you'll experience relief. It may take one tapping round; it may take twenty. For example, "So-and-so looked at me the wrong way just now" probably has way fewer aspects than "the mugging." But even if it takes one or more hours to clear the intensity around "the mugging," isn't that better than living a life in fear of going out on your own again? How much has being scared to walk on the street cost you? A little perspective helps. And remember that one tapping round takes about a minute or less.

7. Emofree.com, Finding Aspects within the EFT Tapping Process, www.emofree.com/eft-tutorial/tapping-roots/aspects.html. Scroll to video session with Dave, video session with Rich.

Ideally, you tap on one aspect at a time until the intensity of that bit of the story subsides, to a 2 or below on the intensity scale of 0 to 10. Then move onto the next aspect that's troubling you and so on until nothing about the tapping target bothers you anymore. If you're wondering how you find such aspects, wonder no longer: As you tap one down to zero, another one will generally poke its head up for you to tap down to zero.

You might be surprised to see how quickly your emotions shift after even one tapping round. Perhaps you uncover a big anger aspect after tapping a grief aspect down to zero. Or you find that after you cleared rage to zero, big tears of hurt poured out but then quickly faded after a round and now you are experiencing an aspect of deep understanding. Maybe after tapping on the feeling of not being able to figure out that all-important problem, you're now laughing at how silly it all seems. Laughter like this may happen even though the aspect you just tapped on is how your life feels like it's ending because you couldn't figure out the problem. Don't trouble yourself to go looking for aspects—they will find you.

Once you believe you have cleared all intensity of your tapping target, you will want to test yourself by running through the issue in your mind purposely testing for any remaining points of intensity to tap on. Poke around in that memory, try to make yourself upset. You will know you are done if you feel neutral about what had heretofore been a bad memory replete with negative feelings, thoughts, and sensations. You have cleared the energy disruption and restored your system to balance. You might even laugh at what happened, wonder what the bother was all about in the first place, or forget you had the problem altogether! Remember the story of Scott's snorting from chapter 2? It's the Apex Effect at play.

On occasion, you might uncover something more to tap on even though you thought you were clear on that tapping target. For example, maybe you chose to tap on your fear of spiders and thought you covered everything because you aren't afraid of them any longer. But then a couple months later in the basement, you see one swinging from a strand of its web and get scared again. The fear won't be as strong, and you won't need to tap on the whole thing again, just on that one aspect that didn't come up when you were tapping the first time.

When Tapping on Aspects Leads to More Core Specifics

Here's an example of how effective tapping can be when you tap on the various aspects of a specific issue. Anita, a 16-year-old, feels anxious about her SAT coming up on Saturday. She names the issue, with plenty of events and aspects under it, "My SAT Fear." She easily uncovers plenty of aspects, including beliefs, feelings, sensations, and thoughts about the original concern. For example: "I'm scared about failing," "I need to do well to get into a good college," "I never do well on tests," "my stomach is all tight and I feel like throwing up," "I feel dread," "I know I'll freeze," "I try so hard but it doesn't pay off," "the SAT practice test I took was humiliating," "my parents are expecting more of me," "my sister is so much better at this than I am," "I'm just not smart enough," "why can't it be easier," "I feel so stupid, like I'll never make it in the real world," "I don't understand how it can be so hard," and so on.

Addressing these details with the EFT basic recipe, one round at a time—"Even though I'm scared about failing"... "Even though I need to do well to get into a good college"—puts you right into the heart of the experience again, which is surprisingly exactly where you want to go. Not because you're a glutton for punishment; rather, you are tapping into the energy disruption for the purpose of restoring your system to balance around this issue.

In this test-anxiety case, Anita taps on these various aspects, one EFT round at a time. As she does so, three different specific events come to mind: In first grade, she had to take a test and didn't understand the instructions. The teacher wouldn't answer her questions, and she got a bad grade. Another time, she remembered her mother trying to teach her math, getting angrier and angrier with Anita for not comprehending the problems immediately. Anita also watched her sister sail through her homework and be praised, while Anita struggled and was ignored.

Interestingly, these stories from Anita's earlier life are core issues that are at the heart of her anxiety. They are the foundational energy disruptions that by age sixteen, have globalized as anxiety about taking any test. What does she need to do now? For the time being she bookmarks the "today' issue of Saturday's test and taps on one of these events and any of the aspects that arise, all the way down to zero. Maybe she taps on all three. Then she returns to her present-day anxiety and checks it. When she has tapped enough aspects down to zero, meaning they have no intensity anymore, she no longer has a fight-or-flight anxiety response. She feels confident about her future and understands that she has great potential. She no longer thinks she is less than her sister. She can now effectively prepare with a clear head, absorb the material better, make the decision to get proper rest, take the time to study without worry, and be wholly comfortable taking the test.

Even if Anita doesn't do well on the test, she will now have more resources available to get the help and support she needs, and she will not equate low test scores with being a failure and experiencing shame and guilt.

Getting Specific with Events Longer Than Two Minutes

Before you start thinking, "I *have* to get this timing right! I can't do it unless my events are under two minutes" I want to tell you that's not it at all. EFT takes practice, as I've mentioned before. How long, for example, does it take a baby to crawl, and then to walk? The Buddhist tradition has "precepts," or simple guidelines from which to live. Each one starts with "I undertake the practice to . . . ." This means it's a given that we're not going to be perfect, that it's going to take a while, and that we'll make mistakes. Keep this language in mind as you continue. Your EFT work is a practice, and practice is never perfect.

Let's try that collarbone tapping for about 60 seconds right now. Go ahead, tap your collarbone points. While you are tapping, choose a song, poem, story, or image you love. Go ahead and tap while focusing on that "love" target. Or just become aware of your body and check into what's happening inside as you tap. Experience your body sensations without judgment for 60 seconds of the Tarzan tap.

What do you do when you have events that are upsetting that lasted for extended periods of time? For example: The fight you had with your spouse/friend that lasted a half-hour; the experience of how your mother had you "tearing your hair out" when she visited for two days from out of town; going to the doctor's and hearing the bad news about your or someone else's health, which lasted from the waiting room through to the news to leaving the doctor's office—about an hour, in all; your partner/roommate consistently neglecting to take the garbage out.

Let's look at the first example, "fight with my husband that lasted half an hour." How could you approach tapping on this? Break the event down into bite-sized pieces. Divide the half-hour fight into chunks of intensity. In this case, four big chunks of a few minutes each, stand out: the tone of his voice when he said something about the mess after just walking in the door, which we'll call "his horrible tone"; about ten minutes into the fight, I spoke about how hard I was trying to keep things in order and he mocked me, which we'll call "so sad"; about twenty minutes in, I hauled out all his past wrongdoings, which we'll call "defending myself"; and finally, the end after I locked myself in the bathroom, which we'll call "utterly defeated."

Each of these tapping targets has a beginning, middle, and end. They are short, less than two minutes in length. They carry an emotional charge.

The event that stands out most right now is the start of the fight—"his horrible tone"—that's where to start. The aspects might include: the look on his face, his angry eyebrows, my surprise at his words, the cold tone of his voice, my disappointment that he wasn't happy to see me, he didn't see anything else I'd done in the house, the feeling of all the air being taken out of my lungs, the tightness in my shoulders when I remember what happened, the hopelessness I felt about ever getting it right.

Sometimes, you may be sitting on so many other past fights that are similar in flavor that you will be surprised at the intensity of your feelings. Be assured that tapping the specific fight events and the aspects within them down to neutrality allows you to experience a huge release of intense emotion stored up from the fight. Release will begin shifting the knee-jerk motion of the pattern of fighting you and your spouse seem to get locked into. You're also building toward a more responsive, not reactive, future relationship.

In situations like these, sometimes all the fights you've ever had flood to mind. It can be tempting to careen toward another tapping target right away, but see if you can stay with the one you're on. Remember that you are tuning into the energy disruption, and while you work on the one you refocused on, you'll be working on clearing the others as well. There are times, however, when the other, earlier fight is screaming at you at a 10, while the current one is now down to a 3. I say it's okay to shift gears for the moment, knowing that you will return to the other tapping target after you have resolved the bigger upset. Most important, keep tapping until you gain clarity and neutrality about what to do next.

EFT won't have you tapping away upset only to remain passive in an abusive situation. It also won't relieve you of all your remorse for saying mean things so you can freely say them again in the next fight, for example. Tapping will remove the heavy layer of emotion covering up your common sense and wisdom.

It's not always easy to explore the aspects or details of upsetting events, especially seriously traumatic ones. Those stories are vital, however painful they are—they hold your life. When you release the trauma and the fear through tapping, you simultaneously transform and integrate those experiences into your being in a way that's both empowering and healing.

So do you need to be searching diligently through your childhood to find tapping targets? Hardly. In fact, in some cases, people just can't take the time or don't have the bandwidth to go there right now, and that's okay. All work is good.

When to Seek Help, When to Tap on Your Own

Please note: because I don't know you or your situation, I cannot know whether you can effectively tap on a significant issue on your own without getting lost in the trauma again. Sometimes you won't know until you try, and sometimes you will just know you are in over your head and need resources to support you as you navigate through difficult issues. My experience is that a lot of the trauma or energy disruption occurred because we were alone, unsafe, threatened, and scared. Having a tapping expert guide us through the tapping process can be of enormous benefit. I personally wasn't able to navigate my big issues on my own.

Would a single parent of three children under age five who recently lost a spouse have the bandwidth to tap on her deep core issues from childhood all on her own? Probably not. But she would be able to try something like ducking into the bathroom and tapping on her feelings of being overwhelmed. In this case, she would want to do everything she could to siphon off intensity so she could get through her day.

Is the person with significant financial issues a good candidate to plumb the depths of his insecurities regarding money? Probably he could use a practitioner's support for the deepest ends and the origins. But he might be willing to take a dollar in his hand and tap on everything that comes up when he holds it and tunes into what it represents. He may also start tapping each time he receives a bill in the mail or on the strong feelings that come up each time he checks out at the grocery store.

Is everything going well except for one little issue that you're wholly ready to work on, or are you super-charged and ready to head into the next phase of your career except for the feeling of being stuck, unable to make the leap? Working with a practitioner who can help you uncover your blind spots makes sense.

If just thinking about tapping on your own issues feels like it's too much, that's where you want to start tapping. Are you too scared to tap? Try: "Even though I'm scared to tap, I deeply and completely accept myself." Do you believe you are too messed up to tap? Then: "Even though I believe I'm too messed up to tap, I love, honor, and accept myself," or, "Even though a part of me believes I can't do this on my own, I deeply and completely accept myself." You could also try, "Even though I don't know where to find the resources I need to move forward in my life, I love, honor, accept, and forgive myself anyway." You'd be surprised what can happen when you take the edge off some of the big emotions.

Now, what's happening when you think about tapping on your own issues? Maybe you have started tapping and now all of a sudden you realize big stuff is coming up. Have your feelings been stuffed deep down for a while, and is tapping splitting some seams that have been holding them in? I don't know enough about you and what you have experienced to tell you to go leap right into the deep end of tapping on the big stuff. I do know that people are all over the map in what they can and can't tap on comfortably and independently without a practitioner's support. As a general rule, it can be challenging to tackle the big hurts on your own, but you know what's best for you, so trust that. You can tap on many other issues and save the big stuff for the practitioner; in time, you'll also have the knowledge to tap on your own big stuff.

When Dealing with an Emerging Issue, Tap

Tapping is a handy tool for when something big and horrible happens in your life such as an accident, bad news, or a sudden loss. You can choose to start tapping on the upset right away; I don't delay when it comes to these sorts of things. Recently, my mother wound up in the hospital unexpectedly—I found out while on vacation with my son. While we were on speakerphone with my mother listening to her tell us what had happened, my son and I tapped continuously throughout the call. We tapped on what was going on for her just before the trauma happened (she'd been at a funeral) and her feelings stemming from that experience, on the many varied fears my mother had, including the fear that the problem would start up again, that she wouldn't be able to sleep because of the fear, and that she could die but she wasn't ready yet. And while I was listening to her, I was also tapping on my own fears that my mother would be taken from me and I would be far away. At the end of the call, all of us, including my mother, felt relief—and she reported that she had no more fear. Her health issue never returned.

I start tapping if I'm talking to a friend who is sharing deeply intense emotions about topics ranging from "my daughter got arrested" to "I didn't get the job" to "I'm afraid I have breast cancer."

So instead of holding on to trauma, you may as well start releasing it immediately through tapping. Are you afraid you'll look weird? It's no weirder than some of the other coping mechanisms people have, and it's a lot more helpful! As always, seek the expert tapping help or professional mental health help you need as well.

When You're Experiencing Intensity and Don't Know What It's About

What I'm about to suggest may seem contradictory—I've spent the last several pages urging you to get specific in your tapping. But tapping is not a linear, logical process. It's a "both/and" process; there's no one right way all the time. Like life, it's a live, fluid process. You may not know what legs are under a big tabletop. You may not know what you're upset about. You might know you're angry or uncomfortable but not why. Sometimes you will only have some uncomfortable feeling you cannot identify. Or sometimes after a conflict or experience with a loved one that wasn't optimal, you might not have any emotions but feel a kind of body ache.

Just tap on what is happening right now. Even though you may not know or are not conscious of the specific event associated with the negative feelings, rest assured they are emanating from a specific event. And you are tuned in, even if you don't have words or understanding about the why of the upset. When you are upset, the tapping process will home in on the energy disruption and work on your behalf. Your subconscious has the location on the map targeted because you are already tuned into the feeling. If it's important for you to know what's under the upset or the big global target at that moment, your subconscious will access the memory of the specific event.

You can even make up an event and tap on it as if it were real. Yes, that will work. Your emotions are tuned into the energy disruption. By experiencing the upset, you are releasing the negative emotions, restoring your energy system to balance, thus feeling the upset for the last time.

Case Study: Global to a Specific Core Issue: Body Confidence

Here's an example of how starting out with global tapping on "feeling fat" led a tapper named Tara to a specific event that resolved many core body issues for her. Tara's tapping on feeling fat led her to a phrase she had repeated to herself for decades: "Why bother to look good? Nobody cares anyway. It's a hopeless case." At the time of this tapping, she was about sixty-eight years old. As she tapped on this phrase, she asked herself, "When is the first time I ever felt this way?" What jumped to mind was a specific long-forgotten event from when she was fourteen: she and her father were going to visit friends. She had been primping and making sure she looked good, but her father said: "Why bother? Nobody will notice anyway." Since that time, over nearly five decades, Tara had never bothered to make herself look good because she felt like no one would notice or see her. She had harbored beliefs of being ugly, dysmorphia (thinking herself fat even though she was a small dress size), and that no one much cared about how she looked. As she tapped on all the aspects underneath this one event, her limiting beliefs dissolved. She realized she was actually in good shape, and her feelings about her body transformed from negative to feeling good about how she looked. After a decades-long break, she resumed primping and caring for herself, relishing herself just as she was. Doing so contributed to an across-the-board boost of her self-confidence.

More on Aspects

Sometimes it may seem like you're not getting anywhere as you tap. Aspects may rise in intensity as you tap and you will feel flooded with emotion for a short time. Let's look further at what may be going on.

Shifting Aspects

Let's say you have your tapping target and that you've now tapped several rounds on the issue but the intensity is still at a 7. You seem to be experiencing quite a bit of emotion moving through, but the intensity is not dissipating. Do you give up? Not yet. It's quite possible that you are shifting aspects, a process that's exactly what it sounds like. You are shifting from one detail to another, perhaps another feeling or sensation or image of the event you are tapping on. Identifying the shifting aspects takes some practice. All you need to do is keep tapping, because the intensity will subside if you are shifting aspects. However, see if you can home in on one at a time, and tap one round or more on each of them.

Sometimes as soon as you tap down one intense aspect, another big one arises. That's okay. Just keep tapping till they all subside. And they do subside.

Emotional Flooding

As mentioned in chapter 2, sometimes, when you tap, you might feel "flooded" with emotion—but don't stop tapping! All the feelings that have been stuffed inside are coming up for air, and this can initially be scary. Keep tapping! It's the fastest way to calm any emotional overwhelm, all the way back down to zero. It means you are wholly tuned in to the issue at hand and have hit an emotional jackpot. EFT is designed to uncover buried emotions so we can clean things up and remove the emotional sting.

In situations like these, don't even bother trying to sort the problem into aspects; your system is literally like a kaleidoscope in these moments, moving through ALL the emotions at once. During the "flood," just keep on tapping and allow the information and the feelings to come through you. You *will* get through to the other side and experience relief. You're going to become increasingly confident about this as you continue to practice EFT.

Once the feelings have subsided, go back and see if you can find any specific aspects that have remaining intensity and tap on them.

No Shift in Intensity

When you don't experience a shift in intensity after a round, it is often the case that you haven't gotten specific enough or there's something you need to tap on before you can get to that particular tapping target. Maybe you need to tap on how angry you are at yourself for not having solved this issue yet. Maybe you need to tap on the fear you have about this problem before you get to tapping on the problem itself. Or perhaps your tapping target is sitting on something else that needs to be addressed first, as discussed in chapter 2.

Other options:

- If you are not experiencing relief, what about zeroing in on a tiny upsetting detail of the experience?
- Sometimes, you may not feel any shift but your body may be feeling something. Focus on your physical sensations, in that case, like this: "Even though I feel really tight in my stomach when I think about what he said to me, I deeply and completely accept myself."
- Or, do you notice yourself getting curiously tired or distracted? Start with how distracted you are: "Even though I'm distracted (or suddenly too tired to tap) when I think about the fight...."
- Are you eating potato chips and looking at your cell phone while tapping? "Even though I need to eat before I tap on this problem, I deeply and completely accept myself just as I am."
- Sometimes, environmental issues such as allergies can be getting in the way of tapping. (See chapter 8). Change your environment. Clear the allergies. Tap your collarbone point. Perform some physical exercise.

- Maybe what you think is your problem isn't *problemo numero uno* needing your attention. For example, maybe Janet is tapping on wanting to have a relationship that sticks this time, but first she needs to address the events underlying her intimacy issues, which stem all the way back to her childhood experiences with abandonment and inconsistent parenting. Don't give up, get curious and poke around a bit.
- Are you just not getting anywhere no matter what you do? You might want to check out an EFT practitioner. And tap on the beliefs that EFT won't work for you.

Childhood Origins and Tapping

The origins of limiting beliefs—core issues that shape our lives, sabotage behavior, and emotional behavior—have roots in our childhood experiences. In fact, studies have shown that the emotional resilience of a developing baby in the womb can be affected by what their mother thinks, feels, and experiences.

I've learned about a number of limiting beliefs from my clients. One understood God to be someone who always sacrificed everything for the good of all. She spent much of her childhood trying to be "as good as God" so that everything would be all right in her family; when it wasn't, she blamed herself for not being good enough. She had a doozy of an early childhood belief that had shaped her life like so: "I shouldn't want what I want, and even if I have what I want, I shouldn't have it."

Another client believed as a young girl that if she would be "good," then God would bring her father back from the dead. When her father didn't come back, she made sense of this by deciding she was "bad," because otherwise God would have given him back. This ultimately worked its way into many areas of her life: Because she was bad, she didn't deserve to have a good career, a happy life, and so on.

Yet another client had struggled in the hard sciences as a young boy after he was transferred to an elite private school and felt he wasn't good enough. Decades later, when he was a millionaire, it still dogged him that he wasn't good enough, which made it difficult for him to enjoy the pleasures he did have. Sometimes our childhood conclusions produce a belief that colors our entire life. We then unconsciously seek experiences that prove our beliefs to be true.

I'm not saying we've all had horribly traumatizing childhoods; rather, most of us have had a wonderful mix of great, good, mediocre, downright stinky stuff, and even some horrible experiences. We're human, and everyone has areas in need of improvement. Even caring and effective parents can't prevent a child from being bullied at school, from having a horrible first grade teacher (like I did), from experiencing a pet's death, or from getting in a car accident. They can't prevent a child from not getting the grade or achieving the goal they'd dreamed of, from feeling resentful at having to share parents with a new baby brother, or feeling like life is ending if the older sister moves out. The parents may end up getting a divorce—the typical stuff of life.

Consider how many children, even in the most ideal of families, are met 100 percent of the time with support, encouragement, and acceptance when they are in the middle of a tantrum or otherwise being difficult? In many cases, it wasn't because we couldn't handle our big feelings. Rather, those around us couldn't handle our big feelings. We somehow need to restore our feelings to their rightful place of honor. And they are in fact not our reality of today; rather, they are just bits of e-motion, passing through. And yet, the hurt parts of us resolve when heard. No matter how "horrible" our feelings, they are just feelings, nothing more, and nothing less. Say this out loud: *Feelings do not reflect who I am.* You can let the big feelings flow through you and out with the practice of EFT.

Case Study: Current Problem Reveals Childhood Origins

An EFT client named Drew was struggling with a fairly general issue: "My frustration with my wife's helplessness and dependency." He couldn't pin down one instance, however, of her helplessness and dependency. "It's everywhere!" he exclaimed. He had an intensity rating of 9 and a big pain in his neck as he shared how frustrated he was. As we tapped, a specific image from forty years back came to mind. As you'll soon see, this long-forgotten event pointed a big bold arrow right at the core of his current-day difficulties.

When we began work, he could only think of two outcomes to his problem: divorce her or have an affair (a good example of black-and-white thinking). As he started tapping on the global issue, suddenly a specific image came to mind unbidden: his father trying to comfort his mother in the kitchen. Drew guessed he was about nine years old at the time and figured it had nothing to do with his problem with his wife, so he continued tapping on "my frustration with my wife's dependency." But the image of him, his mom, and his dad in the kitchen kept coming up. Finally, he paid attention to it, aware that the upset about his wife's "weakness" wouldn't disappear if he set it aside for a moment.

He named the image from his childhood: "Dad Can't Comfort Mom." The story of "Dad Can't Comfort Mom" is a specific event. As Drew focused on this image, he realized his intensity was rising. He tapped each of the many upsetting aspects of it down to below a 2 in intensity before moving onto the next: the helpless look on Dad's face, the numb look on Mom's face, Dad's arms around Mom, standing on the floor of the kitchen, the window in front of the sink, feeling wind from the hot summer day, hearing Dad sigh. He tapped on the different sensations in his body as he tapped his way through the story such as the pressure in his chest, the teary feeling behind his eyes, the pain in his neck.

He tapped on feelings associated with the image: deep grief, fear about Mom and her unhappiness, sadness for Dad at his helplessness, the feeling of being helpless to help, resentful of Mom that she never got better, and more. Now he felt neutral as he looked at the whole image. He ran the story through his mind again as if it were a movie to uncover any outstanding aspects to tap on. Afterward, he felt complete relief, lighter, and more optimistic.

Drew gained a fresh insight he didn't have before. This is a common outcome. As your mind and energy system clears, you have room for more understanding and insight. Often physical symptoms resolve, too. Drew grasped that his own present feelings of anger and resentment directed at his wife were actually leftover feelings he'd been harboring all these years. They stemmed from regularly witnessing the cycle of Mom seeming to be miserable, unable, as Drew perceived it, to be the mother he needed her to be. In addition, his feelings related this father being unable to make her feel better and to what he, as a young boy, internalized as a result about intimate relationships. He made the connection that he had been enabling his own wife in a way that was similar to what he witnessed growing up. The issue wasn't his wife—it was the emotionally laden memories and a skewed belief system about what marriage is about. He could make different choices about how he related to his wife.

Can you see how Drew's relationship with his wife can begin to shift after he releases these long-buried feelings and the insights that came into consciousness—even if Drew's wife never changes? And with just one image in one session.

Welcome Everything That Comes to Mind when Tapping

When it comes to tapping, include the parts of you that you have disowned for one reason or another. For example, harboring of a "shameful" secret just causes the shame to fester in the darkness. Excluding stuff that you're ashamed of is not a useful long-term solution.

Clearing Shame

It's interesting how many of my clients are haunted by what they consider a horrible, shameful secret from their childhood or something equally "terrible" from their adult years. These are, for the most case, things *they have never told anyone*, which fester deep inside. After sharing and tapping on the event in question, these people feel lighter, freer, and more expansive. In fact, many of them can find humor in what an hour before was so shameful and awful. Just because you never told anyone that you stole treats from the teacher in first grade, or at age nine, you didn't report someone for cheating doesn't mean you should be locked up for life—although the shame might have you feeling that way

Another way to make headway when you think you did the worst thing in the world when you were, say, age five, or six, or ten, is to ask yourself if you would think badly of a friend who had done that same thing at that age. Most of the time, you would show that person compassion rather than register your disgust and loathing. Another tactic here is to ask yourself if you know any children the same age you were when the "bad" thing happened that you did. Ask yourself if you would condemn them for doing that thing. Mostly you'll see an innocent child who was out of her depth and didn't believe she had adult resources to which she could turn for help.

Considering that in some situations your extreme reaction is not in sync with reality, you may as well welcome everything that comes to mind about the tapping subject you've chosen. Think about all your horrible, awful shameful thoughts, beliefs, and feelings as though they are long-lost loved ones. Does that sound crazy? Exiling a part of yourself is crazier. Remember, your feelings are just feelings—they do not reflect your true reality.

What's Under Overreaction?

Sometimes when you've had a bad day, you might overreact to a situation that has nothing to do with why you're feeling so out of sorts. For example, you might feel like lunging across the counter at the store clerk and strangling him or her for being slow or for making a minor mistake. The feeling is big. The event that triggered it is small. Are you sitting on some big old feelings of anger? Possibly. The likelihood that you will act on your feeling? Zero. Especially once you integrate tapping into your life.

Sometimes the rage is just a momentary thing: you've just had a really rotten day and as a result have zero patience for slow clerks. Other times, you might be sitting atop a pile of old, deep anger from past experiences in which you felt helpless and things were out of control. Maybe you don't even have a conscious memory of the event, and yet you have now been triggered by this new, seemingly trivial event. Who knows where it started? It doesn't really matter. What you can do is start right there with what's happening right now. That's your guide. Tap on the rage and just let it be what it is.

You might find the origins of the rage you are feeling now along the long leash of childhood. Can the rage be a clue that there's a rich treasure underneath to explore—when you're ready? When you experience overreaction, use these brief moments to tap into that rich seam of feeling. How would things change if you were able to consider them as seams of gold in the depths of your mine(d). Repressing them keeps them stuck. Releasing them sets you free.

Exercise: Reacting Out of Proportion

Step 1. Pick a time when some little thing inspired a big, disproportionate feeling in you. The feeling might be rage, sadness, fear, or something else. I'm going to choose as the tapping example being put on hold for a long time by an automated phone system, and then when the clerk answers letting him have it instead of solving the problem you called for in the first place. You could also choose someone pushing in front of you in a line, someone who was rude to you for no reason, or anything else like this. As you know, you can repeat your setup statements one or more times. Here I include the EFT setup statement three times.

Step 2. Rate your intensity about the tapping target on the 0 to 10 scale.

Step 3. Perform the EFT setup statement, the first part of the EFT basic recipe.

> ***Karate chop*:** "Even though I am so angry about that company's customer service, I deeply and completely accept myself."
>
> ***Karate chop*:** "Even though I want to throw this phone out the window so I don't have to call again, I love, honor, and accept myself."
>
> ***Karate chop*:** "Even though I'm annoyed beyond belief at what just happened, I love, honor, accept, and forgive myself."

Step 4. Perform the EFT sequence:

Top of head through all tapping points, ending under the arm: "Really upset about the customer service."

Other reminder phrases might be: "So angry at them," "angry they don't care," "Angry about the lack of human help here."

Step 5. Now rate your intensity about the issue you overreacted to on the 0 to 10 scale. If it's higher, then keep on tapping until the feelings subside to a 2 or below. If it's the same, you might need to get more specific about what is upsetting you. Home in on a detail and tune into just that. If it's dropped to a 2 or below, move onto the next part of this exercise. If it's risen, keep tapping. If it's the same, then get more specific. If after a couple rounds it's still the same, there's likely something there upon which the intensity is sitting. Ask: "What's in the way of me letting go?" Use the answer that first pops into mind as your next tapping aspect, then return to the original statement and see if it has changed.

Step 6. Round two. Now let's say the upset from the first round is down to zero, but another feeling has bubbled to the surface. Perhaps the person who hung up on the clerk is now feeling ashamed (rightly) about his behavior. He's at a 5 on the 0 to 10 scale of shame. So now he'd do a round on the shame relating to the event.

Check your intensity. Do you carry shame about the event you have chosen to tap on? If so, rate your intensity on the 0 to 10 scale.

Step 7. Perform the EFT basic recipe setup statement. We will continue with our example.

> ***Karate chop:*** "Even though I'm ashamed I let that clerk have it, I love, honor, accept, and forgive myself."
>
> ***Karate chop:*** "Even though I'm ashamed of my behavior, I love myself anyway."
>
> ***Karate chop:*** "Even though I'm ashamed and alarmed at how out of control I just got, I choose peace and I'm curious what the rage is about."

Step 8. Now, our caller would perform the EFT sequence using the reminder phrase: "ashamed at my bad behavior" to tap down the rest of the points until he hits 0 on the intensity scale.

Step 9. Test your own situation and feeling for intensity again. This is your feedback loop.

Step 10. Keep tapping on all aspects of the event until you feel neutral.

....

In the example above, the tapper might be horrified at his overreaction. Then he would tap on: "Even though I'm scared I won't be able to control myself the next time, I deeply and completely accept myself." Or maybe the tapper feels remorse: "Even though I wish I hadn't overreacted like that and I'm sorry, I deeply and completely accept myself." Then he might suddenly realize he was just frustrated about his day and took it out on the clerk and that he should call the company back and apologize. Maybe he will decide to practice being especially kind to all customer service agents going forward. Or maybe he's afraid he's going to turn out just like his rage-filled father, who is now living in isolation, estranged from the family. The point is: Tap!

Stuff that Keeps Popping Up: Core Issues and Limiting Beliefs

You might have noticed that certain themes come up in your life or as you tap. They may be themes along the lines of: "I have to be perfect," "I'm not good enough no matter what I do," "I'm a loser," "I don't deserve it," "I'm not lovable," "I don't belong," "I have to be sick to get love," "it's not safe," "there's never enough," "you can't trust anyone," "I'll do it even though I don't want to," and so on. These recurring phrases don't appear all the time—only when your energy disruption is activated. They are limiting beliefs or core issues. I consider them trapdoors, snares, or even rabbit holes that you step into and then are suddenly awash in negative feelings or unfortunate thought patterns or unhelpful behaviors.

Core issues are like deep themes that run throughout the background of our lives sapping energy, closing down or limiting opportunities, and often serving as the unconscious forces that shape the very direction of our lives. They are the fallout from events that for the most part happened when we were really little.

You may come face to face with a core issue when you apply EFT to a tapping target. You may confront a core issue when you decide to step outside of your comfort zone, stretched far beyond what you are used to, or when you have had a really rough day. That's when the default, repetitive voices that are somehow designed to keep you safe and in your place kick in. The voices that say "I'm such a loser," "it's hopeless," "it's all my fault," "I'm not safe," "I'll never get what I want." It's almost like kicking yourself when you're down, in a way. At the very moment you need a pep talk, you give yourself the "I'm bad and wrong" talk instead.

Core issues and the limiting beliefs partnered with them may be at play if you keep experiencing the same type of problem again and again. Perhaps you keep choosing the same Mr. or Ms. Wrong over and over, you can't stop eating carbs, you can't get the website updated, or you can't seem to get projects in on time. Another clue that you may be sitting on a core issue is to notice when you're reacting to a person, situation, or event in an out-of-proportion way. You may be responding to a deeper issue than the one you're working on.

Limiting beliefs limit your possibilities; it's like having your foot on the gas in your conscious mind, while your unconscious mind's foot is on the brake. You ain't going nowhere till you can clear out the unconscious beliefs and get that left foot off the brake! Examples might include: "I can't go to that college because I don't have enough money," when you don't even check if scholarship money is available. Limiting beliefs are flat, definitive statements.

Here are examples of personal limiting beliefs: "Life is about suffering so you must suffer." "You can't have what you want and shouldn't even want what you want." "Good girls don't do this." "Big boys don't do that." These beliefs may have the words "should," "always," "never," "impossible," and "can't" in them. Do you get the picture? Core issues and limiting beliefs are survival and fear-based.

When you uncover a personal core issue, you may suddenly gain an understanding of the extent to which you've been just coping, what it has cost you, where and how you've been affected, and who else has been affected. You may have the sudden realization that you want it to be gone immediately. Core issues aren't going anywhere when you're in that state of mind, so rather than freaking out, get curious about your core issue. Learn more about it. Keep in mind you may also need time to grieve as you absorb the magnitude of the core issue. Ultimately, once you know about something, you can do something about it. Tap, and you can let it go.

Ask yourself: What proof do I have that this is true? Has it always been true for me? When did I first hear or believe this to be true? What sorts of experiences have I had that prove this to be true? What's the upside of having this core issue or belief? Who would I be or what would my life be like if this weren't true? Your answers will provide you with many different events to tap on.

Please note that you can interrupt negative self-talk or your inner critic, ruminations, worries, and obsessive thoughts by tapping. You can then point your tapping on the specific situation that triggered the thought pattern.

Another way to uncover core issues are questions like these: what does that (feeling or problem) remind you of? What's the earliest time you remember feeling that way? What's the one memory you wish you didn't have? What else was happening in your life around the time things changed for you? What's the one thing from your past you could have lived without?[8]

Allow yourself to go with whatever comes to mind. Go ahead, try it out!

Exercise: List Your Negative Self-Talk and Situations in Which It Arises

In your EFT journal, take a few minutes to list stock phrases that come to mind, mottos from your childhood, things you say aloud or to yourself automatically without really considering their impact.

8. Rue Hass, "Asking good questions to elicit tappable issues," www.emofree.com/articles-ideas/general-ideas/to-ask-questions-article.html.

What proof do you have that these things are true? List any events that appear to confirm your negative self-talk or challenging thought patterns, as you will use these as tapping fodder on your own. So, for example, if one of your beliefs is "I never get things right," when does that belief feel really true? It feels true after spending time with "my alcoholic father, trying to take care of him, like just last Saturday when ...." Or, does it feel true when "my sister calls and I do as much as I can and it's never enough for her?" Or, does it somehow bring up an aspect of your childhood where "no matter how hard I tried to please her, Mom never approved, like that time when ..." Tap out the so-called proof that what you do is never right or never enough, and you'll start to see all kinds of areas of your life when what you do is just right and is enough!

Exercise: Use Your Body as a Tapping Resource

To connect with your body as a resource, scan your body right now. Are you aware of any unpleasant physical sensations? These can include aches, pains, throbs, burning, tingling, tightening, clenching, nervous ticks, tickles, prickly fingers, tight toes, phlegm in throat, nervous laughs, ringing in the ears, difficulty swallowing, nausea, acid reflux, sore muscles, constipation, or loose ligaments. They can show up as: feeling like there's something in your throat when there's not, butterflies in the stomach, gut sensations, difficulty breathing, feeling a heavy weight, feeling sick in any number of ways, symptoms relating to various physical ailments, including phantom limb pain, low libido, no appetite, cravings. What's your body saying to you right now? When you get upset, what happens in your body? If you're not sure, consider an upsetting experience and note what is happening in your body.

List the physical feelings in your EFT journal. Chances are these parts of your body might be storage spaces for your upsetting emotions, a safe harbor or vault for feelings. Use these physical sensations as clues to buried emotional treasure that can be released to experience freedom.

Exercise: List Problem Thoughts, Feelings, Sensations

Scan your mind for a time when you had an upsetting experience. What happens when you get upset? What thoughts, feelings, and body sensations do you experience? List them.

For example, if you have struggles with insomnia or waking up at the drop of a hat, what kinds of thoughts waken you at night? What are your concerns before you go to bed? Are you feeling guilty for waking up your partner? Do you fear getting sick if you don't sleep well? As bedtime draws nearer, do you dread going to sleep? If you are a worrier in the morning, what worry-thoughts do you have?

List everything that comes to mind about the upsetting experience you have chosen. Now, tap on every aspect of it.

EFT allows the free flow of feelings out of a person's system, where they have been buried or endlessly recycled, like in the movie *Groundhog Day* in which the same miserable day happens over and over. Using EFT, we can consciously see everything in our lives as clues to help us fully experience ourselves and reconnect with our true nature and purpose. Whenever you find yourself unable to think straight or act rationally in some area of your life, you might suspect some kind of energy disruption from a troubling memory or event beneath that surface situation.

Review: Checklist for when Tapping Isn't Working

Consider the following:

1. Are you being specific enough in your EFT setup phrase and tapping target?
2. Are you focusing on one aspect at a time? Is it the most intense aspect?
3. Are you giving yourself a calm, dedicated time and space to tap?
4. Ask: Is there a good reason for remaining the way I am?
5. Is there anything around you that might be toxic or allergenic? Try moving to another space, and tap again.
6. Are you exhausted and simply need sleep?
7. Are you in crisis and just flooded with emotion? If so, simply tap on that first, even with no words, before proceeding further. Tapping and breathing relieves flooding within a few rounds.
8. If you continue to feel overwhelmed or out of your depth, seek an experienced EFT practitioner, a therapist, or other professional for help.

In Conclusion

This chapter covered important foundational concepts, including: how to get specific when you tap; how to uncover and address aspects within events; how tapping on one topic will often clear up something seemingly unrelated (generalization); how to uncover core issues and limiting beliefs; how to harvest your negative thoughts, body sensations, and feelings for EFT; and essential questions to ask yourself to find tapping targets.

In the next chapter, we'll put everything together with some major EFT heavy lifters, including the Tell the Story Technique and the Personal Peace Procedure. These protocols offer you a way to systematically collapse the emotional impact of past traumas, large and small, from your life.

Chapter 4

Tried and True EFT Tools to Support Your Tapping

Why don't we replay our good memories over and over again the way we do our bad memories? It's time to put a stop to the endless bad movies. The EFT tools presented here are the workhorses of a sound EFT practice. Tell the Story Technique, the Movie Technique, and the Personal Peace Procedure offer you a way to collapse emotional intensity surrounding bothersome memories (problem stories and experiences) whether they happened seventy years ago or just yesterday. These techniques combine everything you have learned so far to resolve tappable issues safely and gently, minimizing suffering. We'll also briefly cover the Tearless Trauma Technique and Chase the Pain, which are fully covered in chapter 8. These Gold Standard techniques are the basis of any solid EFT personal or professional tapping practice. Over time you'll get the hang of them and call on these techniques regularly.

Tell the Story Technique

The Tell the Story Technique guides you through a traumatic event or part of a traumatic event that lasted three minutes or less. It has at least one or two emotional spikes and goes scene by scene while you tap, focusing on how upset you are as you tell the story *now*, not how upsetting it was when it happened.

Telling the story means also seeing, hearing, touching, tasting, and even smelling it. Tell the story as if you were talking to a supportive listener. As much as possible, start the story from a place of neutral intensity. As you start to feel some intensity, stop immediately and tap on the part of the story that is upsetting. Don't move forward in the story until the intensity about that bit of the story drops to a 2 or below (ideally 0). Then continue telling the story just before wherever you left off to see if there's any intensity before moving on to the next aspect for which you encounter intensity. You move through the story bit by bit, stopping at each moment of intensity or aspect and tapping it down. Test each result *before* moving on.

Vividly visualize the story, scanning for upsetting aspects. Projecting scenes using an imaginary wall or window as a movie screen is a neat way to see the story and distance yourself emotionally while simultaneously clearing the associated energy disruption. Projecting the story on the screen also gives you a way to vividly recall it once you have completed the Tell the Story technique to see if there's anything that is still outstanding to be tapped down. Once you can tell/see/hear the entire story without any intensity, you will feel neutral about the problem that plagued you, a sign that the energy disruption is no longer present. You then experience relief.

Getting the hang of the Tell the Story Technique takes practice. How many people can break a story down into minute bits and recognize the emotional charge on each bit of the story? You aren't used to chunking stories down into little bite-sized bits of emotions and sensations and tapping on each one, which is what this technique asks of you. Over time, you'll train yourself and you can return to this book for guidance whenever you like.

The Movie Technique

The Movie Technique is primarily used when working in a group or one-on-one with a practitioner to keep the issue in question private. It is similar to Tell the Story with one key difference: Instead of speaking the story out loud, you visualize or picture the event on a big movie screen.

The Tearless Trauma Technique

When you believe or know tackling the story would emotionally swallow you up, you can apply the Tearless Trauma Technique. It is a way to avoid unnecessary emotional pain by taking the intensity off before you actually start telling the story. While this technique is most often used when you are working with an EFT Practitioner, it can also be used to bring intensity down enough to apply Tell the Story on your own.

In this technique, you don't go into the story at all. Rather, you maintain a distance and guess what your intensity would be if you were to tell the story. To take the edge off, you can give the story a nickname that has nothing to do with the event. Then you tap on the big problem until you feel on stable ground thinking about it, at which point you can perform Tell the Story.

The Tearless Trauma Technique helps you maintain your power and emotional balance as you process really difficult issues.

Step by Step: Tell the Story Technique

Although you'll find these directions work for both Tell the Story and the Movie Techniques, I'll use Tell the Story as the main example and in the case study that follows.

Step 1. Choose an upsetting event from your past. The specific event should have a beginning, middle, and end and be three minutes or less in length.

Step 2. Name or title your story (movie). A story about how upset Dad was with me when I broke his favorite fishing rod might be titled "Fishing Rod Upset." Falling out of my desk in third grade and everyone laughing at me might be "Humiliation."

Step 3. What's your intensity just thinking about the story? If the story/event is so highly charged that you cannot even think about it or say the name of the story or movie without getting extremely upset (anything above a 5), try the Tearless Trauma Technique first before going into the story. Tap on your concern about even telling the story until you feel calm enough to begin focusing on it. Give your story a code word that has nothing to do with the story itself (like the word "blue," for example), and then tap on your fear of telling the nicknamed story. Nicknaming provides distance from the story's emotional aspects. You may need to tap several rounds until you feel calm enough to go forward with the story. Here are some examples for you to adapt:

> "Even though I'm scared to tell this story called X, I deeply and completely accept myself."

> "Even though I can't talk about 'blue' yet, I am safe and sound."

> "Even though this is the big one, I accept myself and how I feel."

> "Even though I haven't ever been able to think about this without getting upset, I deeply and completely accept myself."

> "Even though this story feels bigger than me, I love myself anyway."

> "Even though just thinking about telling the story makes me teary-eyed, I deeply and completely accept myself."

"Even though I'm not sure what will happen if I do tell this story, I survived and am safe and sound right now."

Another tip for distancing is to tell the story in third person, as if it were happening to someone else. When your intensity saying the name or thinking of the story is a 5 or below, you can move on.

Step 4. Start to tell the story. Start telling the story out loud or watching the movie from a neutral place, before the upset happened. For example, neutral in the Fishing Rod Upset looks like this: "I wanted to go fishing and took Dad's rods without telling him. Didn't catch anything, came home, forgot the rods were in the trunk…."

At this point, I feel a twinge in my stomach and a feeling of guilt—time to stop and tap. Stop the moment you feel any spike in intensity on any aspect of the story and tap on that one bit.

Step 5. Pay close attention to feelings, sensations, details, thoughts, and beliefs. When you are activated or triggered by an aspect, stop. Aspects include problem thoughts, beliefs, feelings, and body sensations such as sharp or sudden pains, sudden fatigue, hunger, numbness, or just an awareness of a certain area in the body. You can even ask about where you are feeling this in your body to uncover an aspect. Allow all of you to play a role unpacking the emotional intensity of the story and collapsing the energy disruption.

Tune in to your breathing: Is it shallow? Coming fast? How are you holding your body? Are you frowning, feeling all tight? These are all aspects. Uncovering another aspect of the event is going to help you experience long-lasting relief from the problem story. It's worth it to mine for the gold.

Step 6. Allow for all aspects! In the Fishing Rod Upset, intensity spikes at: "I slammed the trunk and broke the tips off all the rods." The aspects might include: my thoughtlessness, Dad loved those rods, tightness in my chest, guilt, sadness about Dad's upset, seeing the tips broken off, my boyfriend's laugh when he saw what happened, seeing myself standing there looking at the rods, the shocked look on my face, what those rods meant to my father, regret that it was all on account of that loser boyfriend who convinced me to take the rods in the first place, and Dad's look of disgust at me.

Go with the aspect with the highest intensity first as your tapping target. Tap on that specific aspect of your story (movie) that spiked intensity.

Remember to employ the full EFT basic recipe on each aspect. Start with the Karate Chop point, repeat the specific phrase that spiked the upset along with an affirmation, and then perform the EFT sequence, like so, only employ your own EFT setup statement and reminder phrase. You can also experiment with the fingertip points and Gamut series.

Step 7. Rate your intensity on the aspect you just tapped on. Has it gone down, up, or stayed the same? Note that you may regularly see that the intensity has gone down a couple of points, but not all the way to zero. Adjust your EFT setup statement to reflect the remaining intensity (e.g., "this remaining shame") and perform as many tapping rounds with the full EFT basic recipe as it takes. If you're not moving, then get more specific. What's the feeling associated with that aspect, for example.

Once the intensity has dropped to a 2 or below, pick up where you left off in the story; or return to the beginning of the story and start telling the story again *until* you hit the next point of discomfort, which means you have uncovered yet another aspect. You know what to do.

There may be one or more times when you cannot contain all the aspects in an "orderly" manner. That's normal. You may experience a full flowering of aspects (feelings and sensations) all at once and feel emotionally overwhelmed or flooded. Even if you are afraid of all that emotion, keep on tapping, because they will drop to zero or close to that if you continue tapping.

When Another Event Tries to Upstage the One You're Working On

If another event arises as you are working through the Tell the Story event, stay on the aspect and story you are working on, unless the other event is significantly higher in intensity. Then bookmark the Tell the Story you are working on and return to it afterward. In many cases, when you collapse the higher emerging event, the intensity of the other event will correspondingly drop. This is quite common. Remember, they are all on the same tabletop.

Adjust your phrasing as you proceed with checking your intensity on each aspect. For example, "Even though I still feel some shame..." or "Even though now the shame I feel is at a 3 in its intensity...."

Stopping to tap down each aspect is critical to the success of Tell the Story and the Movie Techniques. Most people are conditioned by conventional talk therapy techniques to "be courageous" and to "be brave and go through it." But when they do so, they're likely to miss important healing opportunities.[9] Uncovering aspects is a way to make sure to collapse a problem at its roots.

Step 8. Test to see if the upset is cleared. Testing to see if you have thoroughly cleared the issue is a straightforward process. Start the story again from the point before you got upset, and run through the entire event again. Stop again at any upsetting place you find, tapping down any emotional intensity, until you can finally run through the whole story from beginning to end without any upset. You might even find yourself laughing about the event, find it boring, or you could have a completely new insight about what happened.

9. Gary Craig: www.emofree.com/eft-tutorial/tapping-roots/tell-story.html

Changes like these are considered cognitive shifts in EFT, and they can also indicate you have experienced a behavioral shift.

Testing and clearing aspects is important. Once you have shared the whole story with yourself or a supportive friend and are no longer feeling upset, try to get upset. This is your opportunity to find and neutralize anything upsetting that still remains in your story. Exaggerate all parts of the story: Make the actions of the characters bigger, the feelings more dramatic, the sounds louder, the colors brighter or bleaker, and so on. Make mountains out of molehills! If you find any remaining discomfort, simply rate it and tap until it's gone.

When an Event Points to a Hidden or Core Issue

It regularly happens that insights you receive after clearing a Tell the Story event will lead you to core issues. For example, in the Fishing Rod Upset, the woman realized that all her life she had been seeking her father's approval but didn't get it or received disapproval instead. She realized after tapping that the approval wasn't about her but her father's inability to approve and accept himself. As an adult, she now understands that she has never given herself kudos for her own accomplishments but sought them from others. She recalls a core event when she was six with her father, sought his approval but didn't get it, and taps on that down to relief. And while this is not Gold Standard EFT, she also takes time to tap positively on the accomplishment of that little girl and uses an affirmation that acknowledges she approves and receives the goodness of the things she does. The next time she finds herself in one of those situations where she used to seek approval but simultaneously feels unworthy, she is surprised and pleased to discover that she no longer seeks approval from the outside but rather acknowledges her own worth. A core issue in her life has been resolved, serving as a critical turning point in her life. Again, this type of experience is a hallmark of EFT.

Sometimes an issue will lead to the understanding of the events holding it in place. Sometimes an event will lead to the issue.

While you read this next story, you may want to tap on your EFT tap-down sequence points, or the finger or gamut points (see Figure 6 in appendix A).

Case Study: Using Tell the Story Technique for Anxiety

Roger came to me with a laundry list of problems: increasing anxiety and anger, and concern for his mother's well-being. I asked him, "When's the first time you felt this anxious feeling?" Roger couldn't remember a time when he *hadn't* felt anxious. "Okay, so when did it get worse?" I was playing detective here, a common EFT technique that uncovers tappable events.

Roger told me that his anxiety got worse three years ago, after the second baby, and after being laid off from work several months, with uncertainty about being the financial provider. I asked him what proof he had that the anxiety had worsened, and he replied that he was recently getting upset even with small parenting duties like getting the kids out the door to go on play dates. He detailed several incidents that demonstrated how his anxiety and short temper were now affecting his job performance and his marriage.

Roger's voice grew softer as he spoke, and he was curling his toes and clenching his fingers. His body was sharing what anxiety and anger looked like. For every emotion, there is a corresponding body feeling, and we all have responsive bodies like this. Soon you'll learn Chasing the Pain (chapter 8), which will help you uncover and release the "tight" emotions stored in your body.

As for Roger, I still wasn't sure where to start, so I asked him what sensations he was having right now as we talked about anxiety. He said there was tightness in his chest and several other sensations. I noted the sensations, and then we started following the physical ones to see where they led. The tightness in his chest was a 10 and he also felt a fist in his gut and a pain in his left side of the neck, but those were lower in their intensity. We tapped on the chest tightness until it was about a 5. Then I asked him if any image, event, or story came to mind as we tapped, or whether he felt this feeling before and when. The next steps we went through are in stages so you can follow along, if you like, with your own story

Step 1. Identify the story you want to work on. A specific story, long buried, bubbled up to Roger's mind. "How long is the story?" I asked. He replied it was about thirty seconds. It had a beginning, middle, end, and a few big emotional peaks. It was perfect for Tell the Story. I explained the technique to him and "pre-framed" (let him know in advance) what to expect from this process: I would likely cut him off in mid-story if it looked like he was experiencing intensity but my intention was not to be rude, only to make sure we tapped the emotional charge out of each aspect he felt so we could resolve the trauma at its roots.

Roger didn't believe there was any trauma relating to this unknown story; he wanted to tap on his today anxiety. I explained that because this particular story came to mind as we tapped on the physical places where he was feeling anxiety, then the story was probably related to the anxiety, even if he felt nothing right now. These little stories from childhood, as noted, can be the cornerstone of core issues now playing themselves out in a person's current-day challenges. Is it a coincidence that the story comes to mind when tapping on anxiety? Nope, it's cooperation—the conscious and subconscious working together. My sense was that Roger's story had laid a big part of the foundation for his anxiety.

Step 2. Name the story. He named his story "The Goulash Scare" and it can be summarized as such: Around the age of six, while eating dinner, Roger witnessed his alcoholic mom throw a pot of Hungarian goulash at the wall after his dad angered her. Roger's physical sensations as we discussed them made it clear that this was a bigger story than he thought. Using intuition, attention, and EFT, everything counts. When you have an intuitive insight, follow it. The worst that can happen is that it goes nowhere. Your subconscious mind doesn't operate in the same paradigm that your conscious mind does. It has a bigger picture than your ego and knows exactly how to express what it needs to heal when you've given it the green light.

Do you have a story you want to work through? Name it now.

Step 3. Don't go into the story yet—check for intensity first. If there is intensity just thinking about the story's title, tap on that first until you get below a 5. Follow along with the example below; insert your own title into the tapping statements.

"Guess how upset you might be if you did have feelings about the Goulash Scare," I suggested, performing a bit of Tearless Trauma and what we call sneaking up on a problem in EFT. He guessed that the intensity would be a 10 if he did have feelings about it, which he again insisted that he didn't.

Using only two pieces of information—a guessed intensity number of 10 and a story title—we globally tapped on the title, "Goulash Scare." "Even though I've got this Goulash Scare story…" (insert your title if you want to work on one). His emotions began to spike up. He reported feeling upset and unidentified feelings relating to this event that happened thirty years ago. We tapped three rounds on just guessing until intensity dropped to a 1, which meant he was ready to start telling the story.

Step 4. Start at a neutral place telling your story now. Roger started from as neutral a place as he could find—before the actual event. The family was seated at the table, just tucking into lunch, and his mother and father were discussing something. When Roger got to the part where his dad said, "I'm fed up with doing everything myself," Roger's voice softened and slowed. He indicated to me that he was also feeling sadness. It was time to stop telling the story and to start tapping on the energy disruption.

Step 5. Stop when intensity rises and tap on just that one aspect. We stopped the narration and took an intensity rating. Roger said he was at a 7 of sadness intensity, with a strange lump in his throat; a 7 as well. I asked if there was any other body awareness relating to what Dad said in the Goulash Scare. Roger replied that the tightness in his chest was back and it was a 10 again.

If you are tapping with this example, tune into both emotional and physical sensations.

Step 6. Perform the EFT basic recipe on the one highest aspect you uncovered. Here's what we did with Roger:

> ***Karate chop:*** "Even though I'm feeling tightness in my chest when I think about Dad saying, 'I'm fed up with doing everything myself' in the Goulash Scare, I deeply and profoundly accept myself."
>
> "Even though in the Goulash Scare Dad said, 'I'm fed up with doing everything myself,' and I have this tight feeling in my heart region right now about that, I deeply and profoundly accept myself."
>
> "Even though I feel my heart all tight when I think about this Goulash Scare, I deeply and profoundly accept myself."

We then tapped down the sequence of points. After just a few rounds, Roger's anxiety over his dad's words went down to zero and the chest feeling had dropped to a 3. I decided we'd continue—meaning the chest would be bookmarked for the moment—and recheck that 3 rating after a few rounds. He started telling the story again from the beginning, and this time when he got to the part about what his dad said, the soft voice and lump in his throat spiked at a 9. We tapped on these aspects until they subsided, somewhat. I asked him what feeling the soft voice and throat lump might be relating to, and he answered "sadness" that spiked at a 10. The chest tightness was also back. We left the chest for the moment and tapped on the sadness about what his dad said. Clearly, emotions were jumping around as the disruption cleared. We had only just gotten to this one part of the story, and already he had released a significant amount of emotion. Here's one setup: "Even though I've got what Dad said in my throat and in my voice, I deeply and completely accept myself." (Note that physical expression of upset is part and parcel of EFT.) Another setup was: "Even though I'm sad about Dad's words in the Goulash Scare, it happened, and it's over now."

Step 7. Tap on aspects one at a time. Go with the highest intensity aspect first. Is anything standing out about your example? Give it a number on the intensity scale and start tapping. As for Roger, the tightness subsided as did the sadness, and he was now feeling fear about what Dad said. Again, we had not gone beyond that one point in the story.

We continued, with his starting at the beginning and carefully tapping at each aspect that had intensity throughout the story. We used the intensity scale as a continual feedback loop to know when to move forward. We moved forward when his intensity on an aspect subsided to below a 2. After about forty minutes, we were closing in on the end of the story.

Like many people, Roger had wanted to run through the entire story all at once. But think of a traumatic story in your own past. How far has telling that story over and over again—worrying it like a bone—without tapping gotten you? In Roger's case, I would have done him a disservice to let him do that. We wouldn't have found all the troubling aspects of the story nor been able to collapse them.

Aspects are like diamonds in the rough—you wouldn't throw one of those out, would you?

In the Goulash Scare memory, we tapped on aspects that included: the look on Dad's face; the angry look on Mom's face; the tone of Dad's voice; the sound of Mom's footsteps; seeing her stomp away; the color of the tablecloth; the sight of goulash on the wall; the sound of the dish crashing; the feeling of being frozen; the fear; helplessness; the need to be really, really quiet; the confusion; and more.

Step 8. Test results. Your event is resolved when you have no intensity at all when you think of the story. By the time we got to running through the whole thing as if it were a movie with deliberate exaggeration, making it bigger, brighter, louder, angrier, and so forth, he was laughing about how silly the goulash looked sliding down the wall, "like a Jackson Pollock painting," he said. There were no lurking aspects uncovered. He still couldn't scare up any upset. His whole body had relaxed, I noticed. He reported later that his short fuse had lengthened a bit and that while out with his children, something that normally would have put him into anxiety mode didn't even register on the anxiety Richter scale.

Clues that EFT is working are those cognitive shifts, insights, or "aha!" moments. Roger suddenly realized that in order to be safe, he had appeased his mother his entire life. His enabling of his mom today stemmed from trying to make her feel good when he was younger so she would step up and be a good parent. He said his anxiety stemmed from having to hold so still while being petrified and never knowing what was going to happen in an alcoholic household. He never knew when things would spin out of control—again. The unpredictability was a building block in his present-day anxiety.

Coping mechanisms like these are common for those whose parents are overwhelmed or inconsistently emotionally available. Codependency and being alert but numb had kept him safe growing up. Contrary to what he had told me initially, he realized that his home life had not been as good as initially described; in fact, the level of anxiety he had experienced was understandably off the charts. He realized that he had never been able to turn to either parent to express big fears. He'd had to put a lid on any big feelings for survival. Collapsing this big table leg had a huge impact on his anxiety.

Over the next several months of our work together, Roger reported that where he would have fallen apart or broken out in anger in the past, he had more patience in his professional dealings, more intimacy with his wife, and he no longer stressed as much about parenting. He was also able to just let his mom have her issues without trying to fix them and joined Al-Anon as well. His body's anxiety sensations decreased and he stopped taking his anxiety medication, which had been nauseating him. He also reported not being attracted to hanging out with angry people anymore.

Important Note About Telling the Story

If you're not seeing results, talk to a professional practitioner for help and support. See chapter 5 for how to find a proven, trustworthy EFT practitioner.

As noted, the Tell the Story approach is not inherently the natural way we think; getting the hang of focusing in on one past specific event three minutes or less in real time takes some practice. In the beginning stages, you might start with a one- to-three-minute story and wind up tapping on another story that took place over thirty minutes or some other related issue that happened over the entirety of your life. That's okay, just keep on going. Keep practicing. You're still getting results (see appendix C for the link to additional video and written elaboration on Tell the Story).

Helpful Questions to Ask to Elicit Aspects

Try some of these questions to help you along with Tell the Story: Am I in the scene right behind the eyes of myself in the story, or am I watching the scene of myself and what happened? Can I even see myself in the story? Where am I in the scene right now? If the story is getting too intense, pull yourself out a bit. Instead of being in the scene, let yourself watch the scene as it unfolds, for example. Other ways to distance or minimize emotional pain while you process a memory is to tell it in third person or come out of the story process altogether and after a brief break, return to the story but start from the beginning again. Broadcasting the story "out there" on a wall or window can offer a bit of emotional distance while you still tap down intensity.

If you're not remembering the details, make them up. Implicit memory is the memory we don't remember because we were too young or because we blocked it out. Explicit memory we do remember consciously. So if you don't consciously remember something, simply make up details of the story for what you are feeling. These memories are attached to events, and it's okay if we just don't consciously remember certain things.

Many people are surprised at the minute details that elicit a gush of feeling and then pass. Your goal is to find the gushers to clear the problem out at its roots. More questions to consider to uncover aspects: Where are you in the story? (Outside or inside? At work? At home? Standing or sitting?) Who else is there? What do you notice about the other people in the story? Their words, clothes, expressions, where they are in relation to where you are? Can you see your feet or hands? Looking up, what do you see? How old are you? What time of day, month, or year is it? Is the picture in the story clear? Are you watching it from inside the younger you, or are you watching yourself from the outside?

When you can't actually see the story, hearing it or feeling it is just as good. We're not all visual processors. Some people's primary way of processing is by hearing or feeling, and that's fine. EFT will work just as well in situations like these.

Signs That Tapping Is Working

The obvious sign is that you'll experience emotional or physical relief once you have collapsed the story's intensity. It won't bother you anymore. You may have a new perspective and insight about what happened. You might feel more expansive, lighter, energized, hopeful, or at peace. Another sign that you have gotten results is that the story may be difficult to recall. You might not even be able to place yourself in it anymore. The story scene might not seem as clear or could even be difficult to see at all. Or it might be far smaller than it was when you started out telling the story and were upset. These are all signs that you have resolved the issue. Pay attention to how you feel after the story's intensity is neutral.

Now let's look at a way to systematically resolve troubled thinking and difficult emotions from past experiences and memories with the Personal Peace Procedure.

Personal Peace Procedure

The Personal Peace Procedure (PPP) is deceptively simple but can be profoundly effective if done consistently over time. It is a systematic way for you to resolve troubling memories from your past, and you can do it on your own. First, list troubling memories from your past, ideally from more than a few years ago going back to your early childhood, including troubling stories you heard growing up. Then tap on the upsetting details of one memory one aspect at a time until you feel neutral, before moving on to the next item on your life. Imagine putting a bad memory behind you as simply facts that happened—in the past. Even just clearing one makes you feel a lot better and provides hope. You can also use your Personal Peace Procedure list for tapping targets as you move forward in the book.

The Personal Peace Procedure can help you resolve the energy disruptions running interference in your life. You may have fifty or hundreds of these stories on your list. Remember the Generalization Effect? You won't have to tap on all of them to get relief. As you tap on enough of the table legs, other events similar in nature will also collapse, including core issues. You might be surprised to see how your life improves in unexpected ways as you move forward in ticking traumatic memories off the list.

Exercise: The Personal Peace Procedure

Step 1. Choose a special notebook or folder on your computer for your Personal Peace Procedure. Set a timer for anywhere from five to fifteen minutes, enough time when you're just starting. You can always return later to write more down.

Step 2. In that time frame, list with a simple phrase or title in your PPP notebook as many bothersome memories or life events as come to mind, allowing a few spaces between each event. Number each event and give each event a title or a name. Whatever comes to mind, write it down, even if you are not bothered by it. Assume random thoughts are coming to mind for a reason. Write quickly; don't judge or think about your list. Once your list is fifty events long, you have a lot of good content to start tapping. Regularly review your list, and continue to add memories as they come to mind.

Step 3. Once you've made your list, rate your present intensity level as you think of each event.

Step 4. Gold Standard EFT suggests that you start tapping on the stories that carry the most intensity. I suggest that you go ahead and start tapping on whichever story jumps out at you. You might start out tapping just on the title of the event at hand, but quickly in most cases you'll start to uncover aspects you can tap down to zero, one at a time. Make sure you rate your intensity after each tapping round. Adjust your setup statements to reflect shifts in intensity and shifts in aspects. Note progress as you go in your EFT journal by crossing events off the list.

Step 5. Regularly review your list after clearing five or so events. Add events that come to mind, and cross off the events that no longer carry discomfort. You may be surprised to see the intensity around some stories collapsing from other events you're neutralizing on the list.

While you are working on your Personal Peace Procedure list, simultaneously create a list of areas in your life where you'd like to see improvement, such as relationships, energy level, career, weight, stress management, or whatever else. As you make progress on your Personal Peace Procedure list, check to see if things have changed in your improvement list. Note the positive changes, and savor them. Since we have a negativity bias built in, it pays to acknowledge how it feels when you have accomplished something or are feeling good.

As you work through your list, also note changes in how you deal with the event, issue, or whatever used to trouble you. Are you thinking differently about the issue? Are you feeling generally more optimistic? Did your self-talk or negative thinking patterns change? Have physical issues or emotions cleared? Have you had any breakthroughs or a-ha! moments? You may understand that when your partner turns on the boob tube (or its equivalent) and tune you out, it has nothing to do with you and you've done nothing wrong. Even the urge to tell the wife or partner or friend or boss how messed up they are may cease and desist, and you'll realize that the important work is your inner work. You will also likely stop blaming yourself for others' problems and not be so hard on yourself, either.

Acknowledgment of Your Progress

You can also acknowledge your progress while tapping down the EFT tap-down points (this is not part of the official Personal Peace Procedure). It's about building your positivity, savoring your success, and exercising your gratitude muscle. Tapping on the positive helps you acknowledge clearing something that used to trouble you. I do it like this:

Top of head: I just neutralized that difficult story. That's one I thought I'd never get over.

Inside eyebrow: Wow! It wasn't bigger than me! I'm okay!

Side of eye: This tapping works and I'm doing it!

Under eye: It feels great to put that old story behind me.

Under nose: I'm enjoying this feeling right now.

Chin: What if I can resolve more bad memories? What if I could clear all of them out?

Collarbone: I'm thrilled to have a tool that works. I love this idea of the peace procedure! I'm on board for more!

Under arm: I'm grateful that I resolved this one story, and I'm eager to do more work. Right now, I'm honoring and acknowledging the work that I've already done. It's good, it feels right, and I'm grateful for this tool and that I am committed to healing. I'm courageous, I believe in healing, and I'm at peace in this moment.

Tap on this one from the top of the head through under the arm: I'm grateful to allow, receive, and accept all the good things flowing to every cell in my body and every area of my life according to my highest good.

You can organize your list in clusters of similar issues, categories, or time periods, too.

Make Personal Peace Procedure a Habit

It takes twenty-one days to create a habit, so consider choosing a consistent time every day for at least three months to tap another event down to zero. If you are really busy, try tapping while taking a bath, silently on the subway, just before you get up or go to bed, and so on. There's personal hygiene, which you do every day, and the

Personal Peace Procedure is your emotional hygiene for resilience and well-being.

In Conclusion

Now you have the EFT workhorse tools of Tell the Story and the Personal Peace Procedure. You have a brief understanding of the Movie Technique, Tearless Trauma, and Chase the Pain. You're ready to go out and practice on your own! In the next section, you'll have the chance to practice tapping on common topics. But before we get into that, let's cover commonly asked questions and suggestions for tapping that give you a real-world picture of how easily you can integrate EFT into your life.

Chapter 5
Common Q & A about EFT and Tapping Ideas

Here's commonly asked questions and answers and tapping ideas that I've gathered over the last fifteen years from my own personal practice and work with clients.

Q: How Do I Know the Right Words to Say?

While I've been saying you need to pay attention to how you word your EFT setup and reminder or problem phrases, the paradox is that tapping is not only about the words; the words are just a gateway to the feelings, and the feelings are what's caught inside in the energy disruption. The words—including the EFT setup and reminder phrases—are *not* the most important thing. Focusing and allowing yourself to experience the specific *feeling* you have *is* the critical factor to release and relief—and even if you can't name the feeling, it still works! Here's some examples from my client work:

> Even though I have to get this right (these words, this setup, this process), and I don't believe I can make progress until I do, I deeply and completely accept myself.

Even though it has to be perfect, I deeply and completely accept myself.

Even though I'm not certain just what to say....

Even though I can't figure this out on my own, what if I could?

Even though I need help to make this work, I'm optimistic that I can help myself.

Q: Won't Complaining Draw More Negative Things to Me?

We're not bringing up the negatives to wallow in them. If emotional trauma and upset are covering up all the good stuff inside of you, that layer of trauma is sitting on your essence. All the pretending in the world isn't going to make the underlying problem go away. EFT allows you to resolve the "negatives" that may be standing in the way of your joy. You stay focused on them just long enough to release the emotional charge. As you release the trauma, the positive—your natural optimism and joy—naturally bubbles to the surface.

Every time I hear someone say, "I can't complain," or "I shouldn't complain," I see a person who could use some good complaining time (and probably a bit of whining wouldn't hurt, either!) When we keep our negatives inside and pretend the feelings and upsets don't exist or bother us, they fester and affect us emotionally and physically.

EFT helps you clarify and focus on your stress and then adds the balancing of self-affirmation and tapping to feel, loosen, and release the emotions in your system. Focusing on the negative is simply about isolating a specific issue or feeling that's stemming from the disruption in your body's energy system.

Even if you know that you want to tap on the negatives, sometimes it's still really hard to go there. Here are phrases I have used in my own practice and with clients:

> Even though I've been taught to embrace the positive and not talk about the negative, I deeply and completely accept myself.
>
> Even though I believe that talking about the negative will bring me more bad things, what if that's just a belief and tapping on the negative actually works? I deeply and completely accept myself.
>
> Even though law of attraction says you get what you think about, I'm open to the possibility of healing what's been hidden and blocking me from achieving my goals all these years.
>
> Even though I'm thinking I'll drown in negativity if I start opening up that can of worms, I deeply and completely accept myself and how I feel.

According to Dr. Bruce Lipton, the subconscious mind processes the equivalent of 40 million bits of data a second, while the conscious mind processes just 40 bits per second.[10] And while it appears that we have up to 60,000 thoughts a day, neuroscientists reveal that up to 90 to 99 percent of those thoughts are the same as we had the day before, with up to 70 percent of them negative.[11] So what's running in your background that you're not aware of?

---

10. Meryl Ann Butler, "A Romp through the Quantum Field: A Dialogue with Bruce Lipton and Gregg Braden," on Brucelipton.com, last modified Feb. 7, 2012, www.brucelipton.com/resource/interview/romp-through-the-quantum-field.

11. Christine Comaford, "The One Question That Is Shaping Your Life," *Forbes Online Magazine,* last modified Oct. 27, 2013, accessed January 15, 2015, www.forbes.com/sites/christinecomaford/2013/10/27/the-one-question-that-is-shaping-your-entire-life/3/.

Q: What if I Don't Accept My Feelings or Situation or Don't Love Myself?

Many people mistakenly believe that saying "I accept what happened" means the bad things are okay. This isn't true; you're only telling the truth, and even if you don't believe it to be true, your subconscious mind hears. The acceptance phrase is speaking to your conscious and subconscious minds, telling your entire system that no matter what happened, no matter how bad you believe you are or how hopeless the situation seems, you are *not* your problem. You are more. You are still here, and you're doing the best you can.

If you don't accept yourself and your situation, the reality of your present day, how can you heal?

Find something you *can* accept or agree with, such as "I want to be kind to myself," or "I love summer," or "My niece, Belle, is awesome." Here are a few other thoughts.

> Even though I don't yet accept myself, I can and do acknowledge myself.
>
> Even though I feel very upset, I would like to love and forgive myself.
>
> Even though I don't want to accept myself, I can accept that this is just where I am right now. (I use this one myself!)
>
> Sometimes it helps to add humor:
>
> Somehow, someday, maybe, it may be possible to accept my horrible self just as I am.
>
> Even though what I did is so bad that I deserve to be locked up for life, I am open to the possibility of a furlough for just a little while.

Humor may not always land, however. Can you tolerate a phrase, or does it upset you more? If you use humor as the last part of your acceptance phrase, it has to bring a smile to your face. If it brings tears, start tapping on the emotions that come up until they subside. After that, you might even be in a position to accept yourself just as you are.

Q: How Can I State My Feelings if I Don't Know What They Are?

For the most part, our culture doesn't reward us for having or sharing our feelings, so it may take time for some people to develop this skill. For example, have you ever witnessed a loved one or friend yelling as they tell you about an upsetting event and when you mention that they seem angry, they snap, "I'm not angry!"

Why do we often not know or misidentify what we are feeling? From the time we are infants, many of us are trained away from actually feeling our feelings. We cry, and our parents do everything to calm us down. It's rare for parents to sit with a young child's discomfort, offering patient, connected emotional presence so the child will learn that having and expressing troubled feelings is okay and that after the big storm, they'll be fine.

Actually, the child's distress distresses the parents! Children quickly learn which feelings are not okay in our family and avoid them to obtain approval from parents, the people who will help them survive. But the feelings are still there, inside.

As you continue to grow in your tapping practice, you will develop awareness of what you're feeling. If ever you're unsure, drop your awareness into your body and experience what you are sensing. Tap based on your specific body sensations. Notice when you go numb. Notice your coping behaviors, which are often signs you're avoiding an unpleasant feeling. Or just start by guessing; go with whatever comes to mind first. Guessing allows your subconscious to work, and your subconscious is always tuned in and will make this easy. Here are some phrases I've used with myself and/or others. Notice that the affirmations are slightly different than the standard "deeply and completely accept myself":

> Even though I have no idea how I'm really feeling right now about (my problem), that's okay; I accept myself just as I am anyway.
>
> Even though I feel numb and feelings weren't even allowed in my family growing up, I love, honor, forgive, and accept myself.
>
> Even though I need to keep a lid on things and that's how I was taught to operate, that's okay; I choose peace.
>
> Even though I'm not sure what would happen if I open up to all the feelings inside, what if it was possible to begin to recognize when and what I'm feeling, and be okay with it?

Q: What if I Feel Too Much?

At the other end of the spectrum, you might be awash in feelings. You can take inspiration from phrases like these and make them your own:

> Even though I'm drowning in my feelings and it's too much, I deeply and completely accept myself, anyway.
>
> Even though it's too scary to have all these feelings alone, and I need to share them with somebody, I deeply and completely accept myself.
>
> Even though these feelings feel like they are happening to me and I have no control, I am actually having them and they are not bigger than I am; I deeply and completely accept myself.

Feelings are flickers that pass through your system as long as you stay connected and calm. As you allow them to arise and subside, you'll experience more connectedness, intimacy, and resiliency. Soon you'll be looking at upsetting feelings as opportunities to heal. If you truly feel like you're in over your head, find professional support. And remember, we're shooting for percentages, not 100 percent!

Q: Do Sensations in My Body Count as Feelings?

Those sensations are feelings; we just label them differently than we do emotions. Get in the habit of asking, "What's going on in my body when I think of this situation?" Do you have an awareness in your stomach, a tightness in your shoulders, a sharp pain in your temples? Is your breathing shallower?

Scan your body to see where you're holding tension or pain right now. Get in the habit of doing body scans, asking yourself where you might be feeling or storing this emotional issue in your body if you were physically storing it somewhere. In other words: "If I *did* have a place to store this in my body, where would it be?"

Everyone has places in their body where they store emotion. You'll soon learn more about the Chasing the Pain technique in chapter 8, which tracks the feelings in your body all the way down to an often surprising root issue, collapsing the pain in the process.

The body is an amazing storehouse: it never lies, and it follows the mind's instructions—both subconscious *and* conscious. You might be surprised at all the interesting things your body is ready to tell you once you start tapping.

Q: Who Does EFT Work On?

Who doesn't EFT work on? Those who don't tap. In other words, everyone can tap. And you can tap surrogate (meaning tap as if you were them) for those who can't tap for themselves, including tapping on animals, babies, for world peace, for people with Alzheimer's, and so on. It works. The idea behind surrogate tapping is that you tap on yourself allowing yourself to guess, sense, or express what you think that person would say, think, or feel if they were tapping, with the intention of passing on the benefits of the tapping to them.

Q: Can I Use EFT on Someone Else?

Yes and no. Tread carefully; start with small things only if they (whether your tappee is a young child or your elderly grandpa) are willing, and don't get in over your head or your skills. Complex issues need professional, experienced practitioners who understand how to safely navigate a person through significant traumatic events. Ask yourself if you can be detached, neutral, compassionate, and nonjudgmental of the person. Can you go where they need to go, not where *you* want to go or believe they should go? If not, then tap on your issues first before giving it a try.

Q: What Is a Tapping Buddy and Why Would I Want One?

Tapping buddies help spur your practice forward faster. They don't need to be in a similar place in their lives; they don't need to be friends. They simply need to be motivated to learn and tap with you on a regular basis. You take turns acting as EFT practitioner on the other person. Sessions of at least a half hour each are recommended.

You might actually want to avoid a tapping buddy who is quite close to you and your situation, such as a spouse or other family member. You might get triggered or upset and become unable to be neutral about what the other person is tapping on, which won't make you a very good tapping buddy.

For best results, agree to learn together, commit to a regularly scheduled time, easily forgive mistakes, keep a boundary around check-in chatter, listen to feedback, set some rules and agreements up around how the tapping buddy-ship will go—or won't go. Review your agreements regularly.

Q: How Do I Find a Tapping Target?

You can turn anything that has some intensity into a tapping target. Just hang up the phone after an awful conversation? Did someone's Twitter post infuriate you? Did customer service lack "service"? Those are all easy, honest, and specific. Refer also to the Personal Peace Procedure list from chapter 4 on finding plenty of targets.

Ask yourself questions like: What's the one thing in my life that I would rather not have gone through? What's the one thing that really bugs me right now, if I were to allow myself to feel it? What's the one issue that consistently derails me?

Ask yourself open-ended questions to help bring you to specific tapping targets and events: "I wonder where that started?" "I'm curious about..." "Isn't it interesting that I reacted so strongly to such a little bitty thing?" These types of questions will open your mind more easily to specific events. Once you have a specific event in mind, determine whether you need to chunk it down into more specific events to maximize results.

Q: Do I Need to Use the Same Words in the Setup Phrase?

I have varied the EFT setup language on occasion in this book and in the exercises that follow, but this is a more advanced practice. When working more globally, or with a tapalong, you will see that setups and reminder phrases often vary from Gold Standard. Gold Standard focuses in the beginning stages on using the same setups. This makes it easier to clear one aspect or event at a time and finally collapse a whole tabletop issue. When you're not experienced, fancy affirmations can get in the way of the work.

Once you gain a solid understanding of the EFT setup language and reminder phrases, you'll see that it's not necessary to always use the same words and that variances and reframes in the right time and place can be remarkably effective, too.

Q: Do Tapalongs or Tapping Scripts Work?

This is a bit complicated. Tapalong and tapping scripts can be inspiring but are not Gold Standard EFT. When you rely on a tapping script alone, you are in "global" or general territory—someone else's. Long-lasting relief comes when you clear your specific event at its roots, aspect by aspect. A tapping script may unwittingly activate a big upset in someone who can't resolve it alone. Well-trained EFT experts who share tapalongs have had years of experience and know well the issues for which they are offering tapalongs. You need to see what works for you.

You might also have noticed that tapping scripts may resolve quickly on a positive note. People can come away feeling quite optimistic about their life and their next steps. However, if the underlying issue has not been solved, disappointment will return over time and maybe a person will assume that EFT doesn't work. EFT works; all that happened was that the tapping script just didn't get to the roots of the trauma. You'll find tapalongs online that might provide a starting point for your own inspiration or for a tapping direction, or to give you another insight into your own issue. Since I'm concerned about new tappers' emotional safety, it's fair to point out that tapping on generalizations can open doorways to old troubles and memories but not provide you with the means to find your way *out*. In other words, a downside to consider is that global tapping with scripts might re-stimulate emotions with no clear or safe directions to resolve the emotional flooding or intensity this can bring about. So, one easy safety precaution is to work with a partner or buddy who knows how to tap so you'll have help if you need it.

Some tapping experts offer inspirational scripts on topics that include making changes, borrowing optimism, having a magnificent day, or letting go of sadness. They provide a boost of enthusiasm, like an "atta girl!" in moments when I need some encouragement, even if core issues are unresolved. Sometimes you just need to tap to feel good. I occasionally start my day with a tapalong.

Q: What about Tapping for Appreciation and Gratitude?

Yes! Gratitude and appreciation tapping activate the part of the brain that's expansive, optimistic, and gives the feeling of well-being. Tap gratitude regularly for maximum effect. It's not Gold Standard EFT, but it can strengthen your gratitude muscle. Even when you're down, consider tapping on being grateful for the opportunity to heal this "challenge." Surprising things can happen when you thank the Creator/Divine/Universe/you name it for even the unfortunate things that have come to roost at your door. You don't need to perform the karate chop and setup statement; just tap on the tap-down points expressing your gratitude. In addition, five minutes of positive tapping just on your collarbone point is a way to foster emotional resilience and boost your vitality.

Q: What Is Borrowing Benefits and Isn't That Like a Tapping Script?

Borrowing Benefits is an observed phenomenon and a technique developed by Gary Craig. In it, you are asked to identify an issue you want to work on then set it aside while you follow along with someone else who is tapping aloud on their own issues—even someone on an old DVD! After tapping along, you return to your own issue and observe any change in your problem's intensity. It's not only efficient, but very surprising. You might like to give this a try sometime—watching someone else tap while focusing on your own issues. It's not as laser-focused as getting specific with EFT but it will help you make headway.

EFT's Borrowing Benefits, or Easy EFT, is different from tapalongs in that you are identifying a target for your conscious and subconscious mind before embarking on following along with someone else's tapping target.

Q: How Do I Know EFT Is Working?

Be alert for signs of shifts. Body, mind, and spirit shifts happen both during the tapping round and after you tap. Although each person is different and you may experience more shifts than I've listed, following are common signs of shifts from tapping.

Changes in your speech patterns: Everything from talking faster to softer to whining to stuttering to whispering. After tapping, you might notice your voice is more solid, softer, or better modulated, or that it's easier to express yourself.

Changes in body and physiology: Broad spectrum of body sensations, from sudden aches that jump all over your body, tight jaws and cheeks, to weakness to tingles, to freezing or boiling hot. You might experience nervous foot tapping or coughing, feel suddenly tired, or have a suddenly phlegmy throat, runny nose, or plenty of tears. People commonly experience heaviness in their chest, shallow breathing, or tightness or warmth in their chest, for example. After a round, you might find a suddenly clear throat or a lighter or relaxed stomach. If you've released a lot, you might need to rest, and you might even feel shaky. All these sensations are common. You might no longer feel tired—you could even feel energized or peaceful. Whatever you are feeling is okay, and the shakiness or fatigue or whatever it is will pass.

Changes in thoughts, feelings, beliefs, or perspective: For example: Before, you were locked-in hard about what someone did to you or feeling that you will never forgive. After tapping, you might suddenly have a different perspective and understand the whole situation with love and optimism. Tapping might connect the dots on some very old stories you could never figure out. You may have a dramatic change of perspective, such as forgiveness, laughter, or the realization that it wasn't your fault or responsibility. Old beliefs simply don't make sense anymore.

Changes in feelings: You can experience a profound release of feeling during and after a tapping round. (Remember, "e-motion" = energy in motion.) Upset and big anger over an experience may turn to sadness or grief, which later resolves to complete neutrality—for good. Commonly, an intense physical sensation or feeling drops to zero. Just keep tapping.

Feeling a profound sense of lightness or gratitude usually creates willing optimism about the future. Symptoms of illness or sickness may subside. People may suddenly change their mind about a dramatic course of action. Laughter and a sense of humor usually returns. Life changes!

Changes in behavior: You now are acting differently and behaving in a more healthy way when you come in contact with what used to "trigger" you. You take steps in your life that had not heretofore been considered or seemed possible.

Q: Why Am I Not Getting Better Faster?

You've read about one-minute wonders in which tapping resolved a major issue in minutes; you hear powerful speakers and motivators saying they can help you undo your self-sabotage or other big challenges through a ten-week course, and when this doesn't happen for you, you naturally wonder "What's wrong with me?" and it doesn't feel so good. Instead start asking yourself, "What's right with me?"

Powerful marketing that ratchets up our hopes with miraculous transformation appeals to all of us, especially when we're hurting. Our vulnerability can make it very tempting to believe that everything's going to transform if we just take this one course or do this one thing. But our great expectations of a course or guru don't usually focus on doing the individual work of getting to the specific roots of our real problem. So let's do the work and find the roots. Sometimes all it takes is one event that lays the roots bare. Other times, it may take five or ten times or even more. You can boost your practice by working with a tapping practitioner. I often tap along these lines when feeling that way:

> Even though I need this to be gone right away, I accept myself and my situation right now.
>
> Even though there must be something wrong with me, what if everything is, in fact, okay with me, and I'm just still working on this? (Note the use of affirmation here.)

Healing doesn't necessarily mean "curing," or changing the external circumstances of your life, whether that's earning a million dollars or recovering from cancer. I prefer to look at healing as understanding yourself and accepting where you are right now, no matter what the problem— because only then can you experience peace, equanimity, and eventually wholeness.

Q: Why Does EFT Work for Others but Not Me?

Comparing means everyone loses. Each of us is glorious beyond measure and wholly unique. When I catch myself comparing, I know I'm triggered. Most of us have grown up being measured and compared. How does it feel to grow up and hear a parent say something like, "You are sounding like your brother—stop!" "How come you don't try out for those sports like your friend?" "How come you can't be more like so-and-so?"

Tap on the feeling that comes up when you are falling into the comparison trap. Who compared in your family? Do you have a specific time when someone made a comparison either favorably or negatively about you and your siblings? Can you list earlier times when comparison events happened? These are all tappables, and neutralizing them may clear your whole tabletop issue of comparison.

People have gotten started on identifying their own issues and taking some of the edge off comparison by using statements like these:

Even though EFT is working for (fill in the blank) and never does for me, I deeply and completely accept myself.

Even though I'm just a tough case and nothing ever works for me and I have (fill in the blank, other person) to prove how worthless I actually am, I deeply and completely accept myself.

Even though I'm bummed I can't be like her/him....

Even though I'm so jealous....

Even though I don't see how I'll ever measure up....

Even though I want what s/he has....

Even though it's hard not to compare, I want to be grateful for my own path, my own destiny, and my own divine purpose, and that I am wholly unique.

It is true that EFT works on just about everything I've seen, but not at the same rate for every person. Persistence and specifics will win the day if you stay with it. If your current trauma issues are not budging, they may be bouncing off unresolved early childhood trauma (a common occurrence), and this is where you need to go. Ask yourself about the first time you felt a similar feeling or went through a similar experience to the one you're troubled with now. Start with those childhood traumas and consider working with an experienced EFT provider.

Q: It Seems Like I'm Getting Worse When I Tap. What's That About?

It means you have big feelings coming to the surface. If you have dammed up your emotions for years, then yes, you will likely experience an excess of emotions for a while.

Who said healing was going to be graceful? Keep tapping, and know that you have struck a vein of gold that will pay off. Healing is a big and wholly worthwhile project, and you are capable of it. Many clients report anger as they begin to unravel long daisy-chains of hurts; have you considered that anger may be your best ally for motivating you to move forward?

Q: What f It Seems That Part of Me Doesn't Want to Get Better?

We'll address that more fully in chapter 6, on using EFT to address self-sabotage behavior. Sometimes we're not 100 percent sure we want to change the situation. There may be a few good reasons for keeping the problem that we're not consciously aware of. "Secondary gain" is a fancy phrase for this unconscious desire to stay just as we are.

On an unconscious level, it may not feel safe in some way to make the change you seek. Therefore what you are consciously wanting is being blocked. EFT helps uncover what is underneath the stubborn resistance. "If I'm successful, they won't like me, or I'll have to leave my loved ones behind," is an example of someone who might sabotage their own success.

Q: Are There Times EFT Won't Work?

Sometimes allergy or an environmental toxin can inhibit EFT's effectiveness to work with your energy system, thus re-stimulating it instead of calming it down. To make real progress, the allergy or environmental toxin must be addressed first. Tiredness, dehydration, or nervous system exhaustion may also be at play. If that's the case, start with what's happening now, not with the tapping target you had in mind. Many people, including me, have cleared their allergies using tapping.

Q: Will EFT Make Me Lose My Moral Compass?

People ask, "If I tap and clear out a bad thing, will I then feel there's no problem with doing bad or unethical things?" Tapping will not make it okay for you to lie, cheat, steal, and otherwise act inappropriately. It will, however, resolve the issues underlying the need to lie, cheat, and steal.

Q: Why Work with a Practitioner?

Having someone experienced in helping people work through difficult memories and blocks can help you quickly access and resolve core issues far more deeply.

Effective practitioners are trained to act as detectives. They can help you find your patterns, core issues, and blocks. They can help you make the connections between a today issue and long-ago childhood core stories. They hold the space for you to feel, and release. They can offer up a protocol or a system that you can work within to step-by-step resolve issues and achieve your goals.

A practitioner can help you more deeply understand how to practice EFT for results. He or she can provide feedback on developing effective setup statements, getting specific, and serve as a resource as you work through your EFT Personal Peace Procedure list. A practitioner can help you stay on track so you needn't fear getting lost in too much emotion. Some practitioners also serve as coaches in between sessions. It's not like therapy, where you go weekly for years. I have long-term and short-term clients: some come weekly, some monthly, and some come for a few times and are done. Some have been with me since the start of my practice and we work when they get stuck.

Making Informed Decisions About EFT Practitioners

How do you know someone is a trustworthy practitioner? Some credential-granting organizations offer a certification after a weekend course. But a one-weekend course is not the same as the knowledge an experienced practitioner has. EFT is a skill and an art form—it takes time. The person working with you must have done a fair amount of "work" on his or her own issues. You would want to work with someone who is accepting, nonjudgmental, and compassionate, yet not enabling. You'd want someone who believes it's possible to heal and sees that possibility in you.

The Association of Comprehensive Energy Psychology (ACEP), Association for the Advancement of Meridian Energy Techniques (AAMET), and emofree.com list practitioners who have been through solid training. In particular, emofree.com practitioners have passed the most rigorous of training. You likely won't go wrong with searching these databases. Do some research to find your fit. When you hear about a practitioner who specializes in one area or another, be aware that it's a specialty but that EFT essentially works the same with all situations. Ask friends for references. Check out at least three practitioners before you make a decision. Most offer a free, brief consult.

Website testimonials will not tell you if you and the practitioner are a good match. Some EFT practitioners offer a free fifteen-minute (or so) consult. I require potential clients to speak with me, as I too need to see if I can help them and if we are a good fit.

Below are questions for potential practitioners:

- Do they offer a free short consult with prospective clients? If not, I'd pass. Skype, phone work, or offer in-office visits? Are they responsive to your email or phone call?
- What is their training? Which organization and which practitioner were they trained under? Do they follow the professional standards and ethics from say, ACEP or AAMET?
- Are they familiar with Gold Standard EFT, or how does their practice differ from Gold Standard EFT? Do they, for example, know how to help a client navigate through a Tell the Story event, aspect by aspect? If they are not trained in

Gold Standard EFT from ACEP, ask how their practice is similar, or differs.

- How long have they been in practice, what other modalities do they have under their belt?
- Ask about location—in office, Skype, phone, retreat—session length, fees, what to expect from a session, what you receive for what you are paying.
- When you speak with them, pay attention to how you're feeling. Are they listening, answering your questions, promising the world, or what? Do you feel emotionally safe? After you get off the phone, how do you feel?
- What types of situations and client needs have they worked with, how many people in their specialty areas?
- What sort of results do their clients report? Do they have clients who are legally willing and able to talk with you about their experience? Does the practitioner have an understanding of the issues you're facing? Clarify this by asking what they have worked with and how they might work with someone like you. While no one can say with certainty what will happen in a session, an experienced expert can give you a broad sense of what to expect.
- Ask them if what you are addressing is within their experience and their scope of practice? You don't want to walk away from a session with unresolved issues hanging out all over. Give them an example of what you are going through or wishing to change. Experienced, well-trained practitioners, in particular those trained under ACEP and AAMET, will know what is in their scope of practice and may or may not refer you to a mental health expert if necessary.
- What is their policy regarding "results"? For example, my policy is that if a client does not receive emotional results, and I define that clearly before we ever schedule a session, they may receive their money back.

- What does your intuition or gut tell you once the free consultation is over?

If you are under care of a mental health professional or physician, consult first with them before you seek an EFT expert. I have worked in concert, with legal permission from the client, with mental health professionals who have made referrals in addition to the therapy they are receiving. When you are dealing with emotional challenges and old past trauma, you want to make sure that the person you work with has the appropriate ethics, boundaries, experience, and scope of practice understanding in place before moving forward.

See the EFT Resources section at the end of this book for more information on practitioners and finding a good one.

Costs of sessions range from pay-what-you-can (using a "pay it forward" approach) right on up to $500 or more per session. Average rates range from $80 to $160 for an hour-long session, and sessions are generally 60 to 90 minutes. Other options include several hour sessions, retreat sessions over a weekend, five to fifteen minutes a day by phone coaching sessions, emergency sessions, and more.

What can you expect after a tapping session? Clarity, resolution, relief.

In Conclusion

Now you know the answers to the most commonly asked questions about using EFT, and you know how to go about finding a good practitioner for your particular issues.

Part II of this book will focus on subjects of interest to most people. These include using EFT to end self-sabotage; resolve stress; find physical relief; resolve phobias; address weight issues, cravings, and body acceptance challenges; and relieve grief.

PART II
Common Tapping Topics

This second part of the book addresses common issues we face in our daily lives. It is full of easy-to-follow exercises and tips for tapping. Scattered throughout the text are encouragements to tap continuously for an emotional breather or a pause for when things get too intense.

Chapter 6 on self-sabotage looks at root causes of sabotage as well as sabotage as a coping mechanism and solution to a problem we may have outgrown. It starts by addressing resistance to tapping. Chapter 7 on stress relief explores how to shift our relationship to the everyday stressors in our lives. It looks at how we absorb stress patterns from our families, ancestors, and culture and how to transform harmful patterns. Chapter 8 offers the Chase the Pain technique and everything from how to tap on the physical and emotional aspects of a cold or virus to strengthening the immune system through tapping. You can even tap to recover emotional equilibrium after a traumatizing accident and aim tapping at serious illnesses and allergies. Chapter 9 explores how phobias get lodged in place and how to dislodge them. Chapter 10, the weight release and body image chapter, offers a cornucopia of exercises and opportunities to explore how to transform our relationship to cravings, our body, and our weight. Chapter 11 explores how to apply tapping to loss and grief, which we all face, without suffering needlessly.

Chapter 6

Self-Sabotage—Why We Do It, How to Change That

Self-sabotage is like a civil war inside the body, getting in the way of dreams, hope, goals, productivity, and joy. One part of us wants the thing we want, but another part of us is terrified about what horrible thing could happen if we do achieve that goal, have the love, make the change.

We want to be skinny and look good but another part of us is afraid of unwelcome attention or vulnerability; the weight has been insulating us since we were little. Is it any wonder that diets only work for a little while? We want to be successful but another part of us is afraid of being smacked down like when we were little and "too big for our britches" or the other family members were jealous. We deeply want a committed relationship, but another part of us is afraid that love hurts and the subconscious part of us would rather sabotage than feel that pain again, so we keep making the same relationship mistakes at key moments. We want to turn our projects in on time but we're terrified that they won't be perfect or that we'll fail, so we procrastinate at the expense of our career or business.

And so the cycle begins: we beat ourselves up for not having the willpower, the strength, the courage, the whatever quality to live the life we want. And then we feel worse. And this cycle continues over years, piling layers of hard feelings on top of already disappointing experiences. This negative reinforcing process moves us away from the insights we need to heal. Our self-defeating behavior perpetuates the cycle.

I write, dear tappers, as a bona-fide, credentialed master of the art of self-sabotage, who has changed (most of) her ways. With tapping and other healing work, I have resolved a great many of them but can attest that sabotage is never about what it seems. It could be carb addiction, relationship explosions, chronic lateness, clutter, or physical troubles—self-sabotage is a protective behavior. And because sabotage protects, it's difficult to change. It is our mind and body's attempt to keep us safe in some way. It's not rational, reasonable, and it doesn't even *feel* safe. But trust that your subconscious is always at work, trying to keep you safe. And since the vast majority of our mind is subconscious, guess who wins?

EFT founding master Carol Look has regularly referred to sabotage as being a solution to a problem. It can be considered a coping mechanism that *used* to serve us but does not anymore. Typically, sabotage includes strategies we learned in early childhood experiences to gain approval, love, safety, and the like.

Knowing that your sabotaging behavior is a coping mechanism and a way for you to get love, for example, may explain why beating yourself up doesn't really work as a long-term solution. You can't get to the roots of a problem that way. Next time you're about to berate yourself, you might stop and instead consider yourself incredibly resourceful, not a hopeless loser. When you start to soften around these behaviors and have compassion for yourself, you gain the opportunity to uncover the core issues or roots of the sabotage behaviors, and then you can tap on them. There's always hope! Tapping is a particularly useful tool to have at your command when resolving the components that hold your self-sabotage in place. But what if you don't want to tap? Resistance is quite common, so let's explore a bit more.

Exercise: Journal List Resistance to Tapping

You'll need your EFT journal for this and the next one. Title this page "Tapping Resistance." First, list all the reasons why you might not or will not tap. Write quickly without giving it too much thought. Your reasons might include everything from "I have no time" to "I don't want to," to "I don't believe it will work," to "I can't sit still long enough to tap." Each "reason" is atapping target that will lead you to uncovering blocks to tapping. Follow one resistance "reason" to the end and see what you learn.

Exercise: Clear Tapping Resistance

Step 1. Is there an area in your life that could benefit from tapping but you feel resistant? What's in the way of your tapping? List one reason. For example, "I don't want to." Use the 0 to 10 scale to determine how resistant you are right now to tapping on the problem area. Write it down. Also note any corresponding body sensations in your journal.

Step 2. Create an EFT setup statement that targets your resistance: "Even though I am resisting tapping on (the issue you have targeted), I deeply and completely love and accept myself." Or, if you're just plain resistant to tapping at all, go with that.

Step 3. Tap the EFT basic recipe using the EFT setup statement you created or my example:

> **Karate chop:** Even though I'm resistant to tapping about this (name issue), I love, honor, and accept myself anyway.

Now, apply the EFT sequence with your reminder or problem phrase:

Top of Head: this resistance to tapping

Inside eyebrow: my tapping resistance

Side of eye: my tapping resistance

Under eye: my tapping resistance

Under nose: my tapping resistance

Chin: my tapping resistance

Collarbone: my tapping resistance

Under arm: my tapping resistance

You may choose to tap down through the EFT sequence points several times before rechecking the tapping resistance feeling.

Step 4. Test yourself. When you think of your tapping resistance about the target or in general, what's changed? Has the resistance decreased, gone up, or stayed the same? Get even more specific. Ask yourself, without judgment, if there were reasons to not change this issue, what would they be? And assume you've got good reasons. List them now.

Step 5. Measure intensity for each resistance reason. If you're a working parent with young children maybe your reason is: "I don't have time to tap!" and that's a 9. And it also makes sense that this working mom of three may have resistance to tapping on her deepest, darkest issue when kids need feeding, work needs, doing, and the partner's out of town. Still, you can tap on the "no time!" issue. Even one 30-second tapping round on "I don't have time to tap with these kids and this work and these demands on me!" takes the edge off, moves stress out, and helps you uncover resources you didn't realize you had.

Step 6. Now choose the reason with the highest tapping resistance intensity number as your more specific tapping target. Create and customize your EFT setup phrase for the tapping resistance reason with the most intensity. You could start it with "Even though I'm resistant to tapping because…" and then add that specific reason from your list. Here are some examples I've come across in my own EFT practice:

> "because I won't do it right," "it won't work for me, it won't work on my kind of issues," "it's too hard," "I don't believe in it," "I don't want to get all emotional," "I don't know the words to say," "I'm afraid of what I might feel," "what if I have to make changes."

Add your acceptance phrase, such as "I deeply and completely love, honor, forgive, and accept myself," or "I accept myself and how I feel about this."

Step 7. Now how resistant to taping that target are you, 0 to ten? Write your number down.

Step 8. Drawing on the examples in step 6, does one reason stand out to you? Ask yourself when didn't you "get it right" or when was it "too hard" or what happened in the past when you made changes? Often beneath tapping resistance is the need to keep safe and survive.

List a time when you didn't get it right, etc. Voilá—you now have an underlying event that is likely driving some tapping resistance. Use this as a tapping target and then return to your tapping resistance and see if it has changed.

Step 9. Now what other specific thoughts about your resistance to tapping come to mind? What remains in the way of your tapping? Aim for the specific events and thoughts, detail by detail, until your resistance is cleared at its roots, often in early childhood.

Tapping on something as simple as "no time to tap" can easily go quite a bit deeper, to a core issue such as "I have to work hard to be productive and can't take a break in order to be loved," a learned way of thinking as a family pattern or witnessed in childhood. Thus the "no time to tap" surface tapping reveals deep, old learned patterns and a new awareness of the way those patterns have affected our adult life. Tapping on the specific memories surrounding the belief unravels and releases the unfelt childhood events holding the "no time to tap" in place and the pattern is dissolved.

Step 10. Now note any remaining resistance you named or are believing right now and tap a round on that one aspect, remembering to test your intensity before and after one round of the EFT basic recipe. Tap for whatever comes up around that specific phrase, and then move on to another reason on the list.

Step 11. Review your original list of reasons for not tapping. Which one stands out, now? Maybe not it's "I can't get it right." Great! You can now either tap on that phrase or ask, "When did I first believe I couldn't get it right?" You will uncover events in earlier life where you "couldn't get it right." Tap on them one at a time. Remember, your ideal "event" is less than three minutes, so chunk them down into manageable pieces. You can give your events a title, and use Tell the Story technique. Continue on this same way until you feel the resistance subside, and instead of resist, persist.

....

Before we explore some hypothetical possibilities, you might consider activating your body's energy system while reading. Consider tapping or gently massaging the collarbone point as you read on. Remember one-point tapping? You can also tap continuously on all of your tap-down points from the top of the head to the under the arm point. You can finger-tap, which is tapping on the inside tips of each of your fingers, including your thumb (see the figure in Appendix A) to locate the points, which alone is revitalizing.

Tapping on something as simple as "no time to tap" can easily go quite a bit deeper, right to a core issue. Perhaps in the case of the person above, after three rounds on "too busy," she experiences a deep welling up of sadness. She doesn't know what it's in relation to yet, but can easily use the sadness as her next tapping target, like so: "Even though I am too busy to tap, and feel a lot of sadness about that right now, I deeply and completely accept myself."

She may realize she's not as resistant to tapping after a couple rounds, and decide to try again tomorrow. Or, as she taps on the sadness about being too busy to tap, some specific past events come to mind. Perhaps more emotions bubble to the surface as well as some tears. But as she taps there is a sense of relief that surprises her. So while she hasn't solved the problem yet, she has siphoned off upset. She thinks about what made her sad but isn't as sad anymore. This kind of emotional breakthrough usually encourages us to keep tapping, and consistent tapping over time begins to have a cumulative effect: we feel better.

Tapping can easily lead us all the way back to unfelt childhood feelings still at work in our lives and our bodies. EFT allows us to work on and release those feelings, proceeding step-by-step through our troubling childhood events. Tapping on each event is like collapsing a table leg holding up our "resistance to tapping" issues. By tapping on the specific events or tuning into the sadness, her energy disruption relating to feeling sadness will resolve. Again, most of the today issues we are tapping are bouncing off a core issue or story from much earlier in our lives.

Forgot the words or all the points? Tap silently on any points you *can* remember, or tap on only one point. Instead of resist, persist.

Quick Tips to Work with Tapping Resistance

1. No time to tap? Integrate tapping into your down time: in

the shower or the bath, before bed, in the gym, even during a bathroom break. At work, you can tap with your fingertips on the tabletop or even under your desk. Remember the famous fingertip points from chapter 2? Just tapping those tips will help.

2. Scared you won't get it right? Tap on that!
3. Too hard? Just one point tap. Pick one point you like and try it for 60 seconds. See how you feel before and after.
4. Can't remember to tap? Schedule an alarm or a recurring widget reminder on your computer/mobile device to remind you.
5. Feeling isolated? Work with a tapping buddy for connection, motivation, and accountability. Forgot the words or the points? Just tap on one point and forget all about the words—focus on the feelings. Persist despite the resist. You can do this.

Self-Sabotage Roots and Safety

We all have basic need to be safe, comforted, accepted, loved, and to belong. Ironically, it's how we go about getting these basic needs met that gets us in trouble. We fear that if we fail, we won't be loved. We fear that if we are seen for who we really are, we won't be loved. We don't feel worthy because once, someone told us we weren't and we need to not be worthy to be accepted. We fear that if we are really great, we'll be abandoned by those who love us. We fear stepping out of our comfort zone because it won't be perfect and then we'll die. These ways of thinking and early patterning set the stage for self-sabotage. The coping mechanisms we used to survive growing up don't work for us as grown ups.

Self-sabotage is often self-protection gone wrong: a part of us doesn't believe it's safe to make a change, so we stay stuck in the old. Tapping addresses this stuff—*outgrown* coping mechanisms—quite well. Try these and get more specific:

> Even though a part of me doesn't believe it's safe to succeed…

> Even though a part of me believes I can't do it, or that it's impossible…

> Even though (I've got this problem)… I see that there might be a good reason for me acting this way; this strategy has helped me survive in the past.

Acknowledging the part of you that's self-sabotaging for perceived safety as your protector will allow you to be on the same team. Working together, you and the "protector" can begin to understand how the behavior affects you. You can uncover the behavior's roots and triggers that set you off, begin to make different choices, and finally, collapse the issue entirely.

So how do we begin unraveling these self-protective patterns that are actually hurting us?

Sabotage and Accepting Yourself

Let's start with accepting yourself, sabotaging behavior and all. Until you bring some compassion and self-acceptance to yourself just as you are, change will be very difficult. Remember, you are dealing with big fears and big needs, most of them stemming all the way back to early childhood. Consider creating sample setup statements along these lines to start developing feelings of self-acceptance right where you are:

> Even though I did it again, I deeply and completely accept myself.

> Even though I am upset about what just happened and my role in it, I deeply and completely accept myself.

> Even though I'm not sure I'll ever be able to make the changes I want in my life, I deeply and completely accept myself anyway.

Tapping softens up the hard feelings around sabotage. You can tap EFT rounds on all the various feelings you find.

Ask yourself how you would treat your best friend if they had done what you did again. Would you condemn your friend for having a problem or support and embrace them in their need? Model the same compassionate behavior toward yourself.

When you have to get rid of the problem behavior right now, this is your panic button talking, and nothing else is going to happen while that panic button is on, including resolving the roots of your self-sabotage. Once you begin to realize how sabotage is affecting you, it can be deeply troubling to your conscious mind and ego. Rather than fixing it right away, acknowledge that you're working on it and accept your situation—you're understanding more about your life and your self, right? Once acknowledged, your panic button can switch off.

Here are some phrases to consider:

> Even though I want this (name your sabotage) gone right away, and I can't believe I haven't resolved it yet, I love myself, and I'm trying to be grateful for the opportunity to gain a deeper understanding of myself and who I am.

> Even though I need to get rid of this *right now*, I want to include all of me in this process, even this part of me that I can't stand!

If You've Got Shame, Blame, and Guilt in the Way, Work with It!

Use what you've got—it's great material for change. Shame, blame, and guilt are the glue holding many unhelpful behaviors in place. When you mess up, do you believe that you deserve everything you get, or that somehow you earned it? When you fall into these common booby traps of shame, blame, and/or guilt, it's hard to get to the root origins—the emotional drivers and energy disturbances—that compel the sabotage.

Did a central figure in your growing up years regularly tell you "You ought to be ashamed of yourself?" But seeing that through an adult's eyes, does it make sense for a 5 or 6 year old to be ashamed of being curious, or for wanting to eat all the cake? Our culture is laden with shame, blame, and guilt. Many of our ancestors also suffered and were kept in line using those same negative ideas. Luckily we can begin to change all that with EFT.

Here are some simple starters for working with these three troublesome ideas:

> Even though I'm ashamed/guilty/humiliated at what just happened, what if I'm still a good person?
>
> Even though I'm so guilty for making that mistake again, what if I could offer some compassion instead, since beating myself up has never worked.
>
> Even though I feel really ashamed of myself for messing up again, would I be so hard on my friend or partner if they had "fallen off the wagon" again?
>
> Even though I'm hearing Mom/Dad/the teacher's voice saying "You ought to be ashamed of yourself" or "Shame on you," I choose to be proud and love that younger me.
>
> Even though I messed up again, I am still a good person, worthy of love, respect, care, and compassion.

General as they are, these phrases are starting points for you.

Make Your Self-Talk Work for You

Tune into a specific area of your life that you are currently sabotaging. Listen for those negative thoughts, the inner critic, the constant self-talk in the background. They are there; we have up to 60,000 thoughts a day and a majority of these can be negative. Here's some examples to get you started: *I can't do that. It will never work. Who do I think I am? Why would they pick me? I'm not good enough. What if they see me and know the truth?* Use these negative self-talk phrases to create your tapping setup statements. Write the crazy things that you think and tell yourself, take a look at the list—it might be enough to bring back sanity. Tap on them. Pretend you are an anthropologist from some planet far away in the galaxy, studying the foreign culture of You. Get really curious.

Focus on What's Right

Focusing on what's wrong, not what's right, isn't just a family issue, it's a cultural issue, and probably a biological one, as well. We were made to survive, with a 24/7 survival radar looking for dangerous situations—in other words, what's wrong. Compensate by noting what's right. It takes half a second to notice and memorize what's wrong, compared with twelve seconds to absorb something good or positive. So savor the positives, even if it's as simple as a kind word a stranger said, a beautiful photograph, you name it. You'll find that focusing on what's "right" is a lot easier on you, while beating yourself up merely locks the problem in more completely. Consider creating a gratitude journal, and take your time to write what you appreciate and are grateful for every day in your life. Remember to be positive in simple ways, such as letting someone else go first in line, smiling, expressing gratitude every time something feels good during your day, and expressing thankfulness for opportunities to heal and learn when things don't go so well in your day. And don't forget to tap—you build your good, appreciation, gratitude, and happy muscle by exercising it many times a day.

Who Else in My Family Does This?

You might ask: *Who else did I see beating themselves up? About what?* Do you believe you have inherited this issue so you can't possibly change? Start tapping on a belief that may feel real but isn't true. Try tapping on any early childhood events where you witnessed a loved one feeling hopeless or being too hard on him or herself.

Explore Your Beliefs Relating to Your Own Self-Sabotage

It's common for people to believe it's impossible to change old, ingrained habits and patterns. But what if that itself is simply a belief and not what's true? Could it be that you learned to be a certain way, to be accepted as part of the family system? Is there a time you can remember that you weren't "this way"—scattered, overweight, or unable to ask questions or stand up for yourself?

What's underneath the "it's just the way I am," for you?

Childhood Origins of Sabotage

Children under the age of seven typically view their parents as all-powerful, and if anything is wrong, they quickly take on the blame rather than looking at their parents with a critical eye. To survive, children quickly learn survival skills within their family in order to get what they need—love, acceptance, and approval. Children quickly absorb belief systems and ways of behaving that may cover up the core of their being in attempts to get what they need. But those unexpressed hidden feelings don't go away until they're finally acknowledged.[12]

With EFT, we begin to tap on these old beliefs, and you have far more control over your emotions and thoughts than you think.

---

12. Josh Korda and George Haas, "On the Roots of the False Self and a Return to Authenticity," Podcast on Dharmapunxnyc.com, last modified August 13, 2014, www.dharmapunxnyc.com/blog/2014/8/13/2fdz0k3fs5y5vuv5bjfa6xzp97h6iq.

Get Curious About Your Beliefs; Tap on Whatever Resonates

What proof do you have that things have to be the way they are? Is it true for other people or just you? Is it logically true or does it feel like an emotional truth? It's time for a belief reboot of your system.

Here are some sample phrases about change fears:

> Even though I don't believe it's possible to change, I believe I can accept myself and how I feel.
>
> Even though I believed I had to be perfect for things to be okay....
>
> Even though I believed I wouldn't be loved if I didn't do what she wanted....
>
> Even though a part of me believes that I can't do it, and will never be successful....
>
> Even though it's not okay to ask questions, because she might get upset....
>
> Even though I don't rock the boat because all hell would break loose and then it would all be my fault....
>
> Even though nothing I did was ever good enough....
>
> Even though I shouldn't want what I want and don't deserve to have it anyway,....

Imagine Life Differently

You have far more control over your emotions and thoughts than you may believe. Ask yourself what would happen if you did make a change, and begin to look at your fears framed that way. What happened when you made a change before? What's in the way of you making this change? What's the upside of staying the same way? What's the downside of making a change? What does this resistance remind you of? What's the earliest time you felt this type of resistance to change? Where in your life do you sabotage the most?

Your answers can be easily turned into tapping targets. Where in your life do you sabotage? Take out your EFT journal, and list the areas of your life where you sabotage most often. What is it that brings on the sabotage? Review the last time you sabotaged and ask yourself what was happening just before it happened.

Tapping into these feelings and subconscious rules will reveal a progression of thoughts and lead to options for change, which can feel scary. Change often doesn't feel safe, but patiently tapping will soothe negative feelings and reveal surprising insights. Often hesitance is not about the issue we initially assumed but about areas we've neglected and feelings we've repressed for years.

You can tell you've got black-and-white thinking about an issue in your life when you ask yourself: What will happen if I do change? Take that answer and ask yourself the same question again: What will happen then? And keep on asking the same question about what will happen. You will find that after about three or four "what will happens," the answer will likely be something like "I'll die and be all alone," or "I'll be isolated and revealed for the fraud I am," or "I'll never go out again," or something extremely melodramatic. Take note—you're not working with a logical mind here but the need to process emotions.

Conflict: People who Simultaneously Want and Don't Want to Get Better

Sometimes there are very good practical reasons for keeping a situation just as it is, although we're not consciously aware of them. "Secondary gain" is the fancy term for the unconscious desire to stay just as we are. Simply put, there is some benefit you're not yet aware of, that makes it seem safer to keep the problem. Consciously thinking we want one thing while unconsciously not feeling safe to have what we want keeps us stuck. EFT helps uncover what is underneath this stubborn resistance. If you had to guess at a reason you're finding resistance, what would it be? What are the upsides *and* the downsides of making the change you say you want?

Self-Sabotage Q & A Review

1. Which area of your life do you most often sabotage? Choose one specific area of sabotage at a time and work through these questions. Your answers will uncover a boatload of tapping targets. What's your earliest memory of feeling this way? Does this feeling remind you of anything?
2. When does the self-sabotage happen? Your answer will give you targets.
3. What are the feelings associated with the sabotage?
4. What kind of self-talk do you have doing this?
5. What specifically triggers your self-sabotage?
6. What else was happening in your life at the time of the sabotage?
7. What could your sabotage behavior be protecting you from?
8. What's the upside of allowing this sabotage behavior to continue? What's the downside of changing it?
9. How would your life be different if you eliminated self-sabotage in this area of your life?
10. Imagine life free of the sabotage.

Answers to these questions provide you with specific tapping targets relating to your sabotage area. Remember to stay focused on one target, event, or aspect at a time. This will help you clear intensity from specific events or table legs holding up the sabotage tabletop in a comprehensive, efficient, effective manner. Rate your intensity before tapping, then recheck it after each tapping round, uncovering any hanging aspects. See the progress you are making before moving on. If you still have questions about getting specific, review chapter 3 for guidance. And of course if you believe tackling this on your own might be a bit much, get the professional support you need from a trustworthy EFT practitioner.

Exercise: Imagine Better

Try offering your sabotage behavior a little vacation. Send it to the most special, loving, wondrous place you can imagine, and let it know it can come back after a little while. Allow yourself to experience how would it feel if the self-sabotage behavior was really gone. What would happen specifically if your projects were in on time, you had the job of your dreams, the relationship that fostered intimacy, the body confidence no matter what your weight, the money for the new business, the recognition for your work, or whatever it is you need? How would it feel waking up without the sabotage behavior? What would a morning look like? How would it feel in your body? What things would change in your life? What would be different about how you felt about yourself? How would your life change? Imagine what your day would look like. Use all senses, including sight, sound, taste, touch, and don't forget smell.

Releasing resistance. Note any resistance to these musings in your EFT journal, as you imagine living free of the sabotage behavior; note all the "yes-buts" that come to mind. You can then tap on these one at a time as you are able.

Repeat this exercise regularly. Envisioning life without the sabotage will help you dissolve the sabotaging behavior, reinforcing the possibility of change.

In Conclusion

We have explored the many facets of self-sabotage as well as how to uncover your sabotage areas and zap them with EFT. As you dismantle the underpinnings of your sabotage, you will see real possibilities for changing your choices and patterns. With a bit of patience, honesty, persistence, and the courage that resides within you, your self-sabotage *will* resolve, and you'll see its effect in areas of your life you can't even yet imagine.

In the next chapter we will explore stress. It's part of life, right? But do we have to suffer? Perhaps we can put stress to use for our benefit.

Chapter 7

Tapping for Relief from Stress and Being Overwhelmed

Is your stress dial stuck on high? In this chapter you'll lower the stress dimmer switch or shut the stress alert off entirely until you truly need it. If you're feeling stressed even reading about stress, how about tapping? You can choose one point or continuously tap on the tap-down points (top of the head through under the arm), the Tarzan point, or continuously on the finger points as you read through this chapter.

It's not that we want stress to disappear from the face of the planet; the paradox of stress is that it is a necessary part of the fabric of our lives. It has helped us adapt and evolve as a species. We were shivering cold back in the day; inspired by stress we then created fire. Stress tells us we're in danger and has saved many a prehistoric ancestor's neck. Nowadays, when we *respond* to stress instead of react and freak out, its presence can motivate us to invent ways to make our lives work better. Stress can help us be flexible and adaptive in our responses. "Respond" here means to be flexible and responsive. It's like having joints that allow us to bounce and pivot easily. "React," by contrast, means frozen in place, more prone to injury.

Stress is a given, so it's how we handle stressful situations that makes a difference. When stress gets to us, the same situation we handled easily yesterday can feel overwhelming today. When we are consistently reacting to stressful situations instead of responsive to them, we lose perspective and the stress button gets stuck in the On position. A constant state of stress can become a normal way of life for many who are living twenty-first-century lifestyles, but our bodies don't like it.

Scientists have confirmed the link between stress and illness; 85 percent of all disease is linked to an emotional stress component. Stress drives anxiety, compulsions, adrenal burnout, and even weight gain. Our bodies take so much before they say, "Okay! Enough!" Let's dissipate the disruptions in our energy system caused by stress before they turn into physical ailments. Are you tapping yet?

Exercise: Global Stress Release

Does reading about stress…stress you out? Tap on that before you read on. "Even though reading about stress stresses me out, I deeply and completely accept myself." We're going to aim EFT at releasing global stressors in our lives. This particular exercise is an alternative to the traditional EFT model. See what you think.

Stress Relief, Part 1

Step 1. How stressed are you or how stressful is your life right now on the 0 to 10 scale? Write your number down in your EFT journal. Even if you are not feeling any stress right now, borrow someone else's stress and help them out by tapping anyway. Or pick something specific that does stress you out and rate its intensity.

Step 2. Karate chop continuously while expressing an EFT setup statement one or more times that portrays how stressful stress is to you. Here's an example for you to customize:

"Even though I'm stressed out (or "my life stresses me out"), I deeply and completely accept myself."

Now tap the EFT sequence or the points with this reminder phrase, starting with the top of the head, ending with the under-the-arm point: "I'm stressed! Life is stressful!" Run this EFT sequence a few times until you notice a difference in your level of intensity.

Step 3. What does your stress-o-meter say now? Take note of the level of your stress on the 0 to 10 scale again. Note any differences in your number. If your level of stress continues to be above 4, tap another two or three rounds until the level subsides to below 4. If something specific about your stress comes to mind as you tap, note the specific issue and create an EFT setup statement. Tap through the EFT basic recipe on that issue before moving to step 4 of this exercise.

Step 4. This next EFT setup statement is a reframe, where you restate the problem in a way that is more optimistic, giving you a different perspective from which to consider the issue. Reframes work when the person tapping is ready to receive them. Otherwise, they bounce off like a ball.

Express your EFT setup phrase aloud one to three times while karate chopping on the side of the hand:

"Even though I'm stressed, what if this chapter has some stress-dissolving techniques for me that ease my stress?"

Step 5. One round from top of head through the points:

Top of head: I'm stressed!

Inside eyebrow: This stress.

Side of eye: Too much stress.

Under eye: My body on stress.

Under nose: All the stress in my life.

Chin: Too much stress.

Collarbone: Ugh, stress.

Under arm: I hate it and I want it to go away!

Step 6. Perform the EFT sequence (the tap-down points) using the following variations for the reminder phrase or your own version.

Top of head: Is it possible this stress-busting tool will work for me?

Inside eyebrow: No way! How's this tapping gonna relieve my stress?

Side of eye: Ghostbusters worked for ghosts. What about stress busters? Is it possible that there are some stress-busting tools for me?

Under eye: Could there be ways for me to ease my stress load?

Under nose: Nah, that would be too easy.

Chin: What if it's easier than I think, and all my thoughts, doubts, fears, and guilts are making it harder? What if this tapping actually helps relieve the way I react to stress?

Collarbone: It would feel so great to release some of this stress.

Under arm: I'd have more patience with the [kids, dogs, spouse, work, colleagues], I'd have more energy, I'd sleep better, I'd like myself better and feel better about my life.

Stress Relief, Part 2

Step 1. List the stressors in your life and jot them down in your EFT journal. Now how stressed are you about stress? Rate your stress on the 0 to 10 scale and write the number down.

Step 2. Perform the EFT basic recipe. Create a setup statement that characterizes how stressed you feel about all the stressors in your life. Express your EFT setup statement aloud one or more times while karate chopping continuously, such as:

> Even though I have way too much stress in my life, I deeply and completely love, honor, and accept myself.

Even though I'm stressed, and I've got good reason to be stressed out, I'm still a good person, and I accept myself and how I feel.

Tap down the points:

Top of head: I'm stressed out. Even reading about stress stresses me out!

Inside eyebrow: I've got too much to do!

Side of eye: Ugh...all this stress!

Under eye: There's just way too much stress in my life. I've got....(list your stressors or select a few that fit and make each stressor a different point on the EFT sequence. You can repeat a couple of sequences: needy kids, needy spouse, needy parent, needy dog, my demanding work, the crazy commute, my weight, my crazy boss, the merger, my kids' puppy that won't stop chewing everything, lack of money, all the bills, all my unfinished projects, the dirty laundry, nobody listens to me, what if I don't get well, this messy house, stressed people all around me, all those emails....)

Under nose: All this stress. I'm tired thinking about it.

Chin: All this stress is exhausting me. I should be able to figure it out.

Collarbone: I should be able to handle all this stress. What's wrong with me?

Under arm: Too much stress, I can't handle it all. What if all this stress makes me sick? I've got too much stress and can't handle it all. Help!

See how a person can let their fears run awayinto a horrible future scenario? Time to put a stop to negative musings.

Step 3. You already know that to get to the bottom of the stress and have long-lasting relief, you need to uncover the specifics holding up your stress. But here we'll try another tapping sequence, a variation on Gold Standard EFT, starting at the top-of-the-head point. This is a more global approach to stress. You'll notice that the words vary, but the concept of *stressed out* is the same. See what comes up for you as you follow along. Here's the **second tapping sequence, two rounds:**

Top of head: I'm so stressed out. I wish I knew how to manage my life better.

Inside eyebrow: Other people manage stress so maybe I can, too.

Side of eye: But I don't know how—yet. There's too much going on all the time! I haven't learned how to ease up when I feel like this.

Under eye: The stress doesn't really work for me. I feel tight all over. That's making it worse!

Under nose: I wonder how I can relax and be peaceful, even with all the stressful demands on me. When I'm calm, things go smoother, stress goes away, I'm more energized.

Chin: Is it even possible to be calm with all this crazy stress in my life?

Collarbone: Probably. It's not a saber-toothed tiger is not chasing me; I just have some stress, is all.

Under arm: I wonder how it would feel to relax, even with everything I have to do and all my to-do lists. Wow. What a great idea. I could breathe fully and deeper, relax my body. I might even think more clearly. Maybe everything wouldn't be an emergency anymore.

Top of head: What if I could relax and be peaceful instead of anticipating all the stress? That would be a relief!

Inside eyebrow: What if stress was actually an invitation to calm down, get centered, and ground?

Side of eye: No more freaking out about the day and the demands on my life. Wonder if that would make a difference.

Under eye: It feels so good to be calm and centered, no matter what's going on around me. I am grounded, calm, and peaceful.

Under nose: I breathe more fully, feel more connected, good. Not get all stuck in my head.

Chin: My body relaxes. I am more connected to myself, to others, and to life. I see my possibilities and experience well-being.

Collarbone: Everything flows more smoothly from here.

Under arm: Tension flows like a gentle stream right out of me. I love that idea. I love feeling peaceful, relaxed, and grounded.

Step 4. Now, check back in on your stress level. Has it changed? Any insights? If you are still above 3 on the 0 to 10 scale, tune in to one very specific stressor and tap on all aspects relating to that one stressor in your life. Even if your "stress" is now just a few points lower, you have made headway!

....

But what if your intensity remains really high?

When You Can't Tap It Down

What do you do when you are unable to resolve the stress or any other issue at its roots? In the exercise above, we worked globally on stress to ideally take the edge off, but if you get caught in a situation where the intensity is high, you don't know how to go further. You feel lost or like there isn't time. You can box up your issue, and I'll show you how right now. You can also seek professional support that can help you navigate toward calmer waters.

....

Exercise: Box Up Your Stress (or Upset) for Now

We don't always have the time to resolve our problems down to zero. Sometimes they refuse to budge. Rather than walk around feeling like a basket case, you can box up the stress or upset and set it aside so you can get back to your life for now.

Here's something that I offer my clients: spread your arms wide and scoop the stress or the upset from all around your body into a little ball. Got it? Now, choose a receptacle to store this issue in just for now so you can continue with your life. Would you like to box it up as a present? A treasure chest or jewelry box? Store it in the compost heap or in your back pocket?

Tap down the points

Top of head: I'm closing all the doors and windows I opened—for now.

Inside eyebrow: It's time to set this issue aside for now, in a safe place for me and the stress.

Side of eye: I'm storing you right here in this treasure chest (or name your storage space).

Under nose: I know just where you are. And I don't have to do a thing right now.

Chin: You can do your work on my behalf while I go about my day.

Collarbone: Releasing all thoughts, images, upsets, and body feelings related to the stress into this box.

Under arm: Setting this box aside for now. Closing all doors and windows on this work. Letting it all go. I am safe. I am loved. I am healing. I don't have to do anything. I can just relax, and breathe. I choose to let go and store all of this upset in this box There's plenty of room and plenty of time. Letting it all go for now. I can always call this back when I have the time, energy, and will. For now, it will do its work on my behalf, and I don't need to do a thing.

Now breathe in, allowing your out-breath to extend at least twice as long as your in-breath. This long breathing on the exhale signals to the body that it's time to relax.

Another Stress Buster

Try Dr. Andrew Weil's 4-7-8 quick breathing exercise that helps the body slip from the sympathetic nervous system (fight-flight) to the parasympathetic (eat-sleep-breathe). Inhale through your nose to the count of four, hold your inhale gently to the count of seven, and then open your mouth and take a long sigh out to the count of eight. Repeat four times, and you'll relax.[13]

How Stress Affects the Body, Working with the Body to Relieve Stress

When you are upset, angry, or scared, your body correspondingly creates a biochemical response that reflects the emotion you are experiencing. How does the stress response look and feel? The body contracts, breathing is shallow, digestion gets tight, and the hormone cortisol is released. Muscles get tight, jaws clench, joints stiffen, and we don't feel good.

You may not feel the effect of stress on your body at first, but as you begin to pay attention to the sensations in your body under stress, your body will show you where it holds it. The most common storage space seems to be the back.[14] Other common places people report stress being held are where they've had injuries such as from a car accident, sprain, or strain; in the gut; or in tight shoulders or neck.

13. Andrew Weil, M.D., "The 4-7-8 Breath: Health Benefits and Demonstration," Accessed January 11, 2015, www.drweil.com/drw/u/VDR00112/The-4-7-8-Breath-Benefits-and-Demonstration.html.

14. "Back Pain," Accessed January 11, 2015, www.nlm.nih.gov/medlineplus/backpain.html.

When you are feeling an unpleasant sensory (or body) experience, ask yourself, "What's happening right now? Am I aware of something that is upsetting me emotionally? What just happened right before I started feeling blah in my body?"

Tapping on your body sensations alone is often enough to relieve stress. Your body's sensory information is your cue to take a moment to tap, slow down, and breathe. Mindfully breathing brings awareness to your whole body. Start noticing and your body will reveal its secrets. Your body is designed to be in healthy, wholesome partnership with you.

When stress is present, we're in a state of contraction—unlikely to step outside of our comfort zone, think clearly through a conflict, avoid the late-night carb binge, or make headway on other goals. We're more likely to blame, shame, feel sorry for ourselves, and ask ourselves one of those never-ending, non-helpful questions such as "Why me?!" We're not in the neocortex, the part of our brain that allows for creative and abstract thinking and resourceful problem-solving. We're in the part of the brain that feels like the end of the world is near.

When we feel loving, secure, grounded, or happy, our corresponding biochemical make us feel expansive, healthy, light, and good. We feel like doing the things we love. Life flows effortlessly. During these times, we easily achieve our goals. Truly, our bodies can't help but reflect our thoughts and emotions; they're designed to do so! Which state of mind do you prefer—reactive or responsive?

With EFT, we shift the way we respond to stressful situations in our lives. When we stay grounded and centered in the face of stress, the stress hormones in our body are not activated: Adrenalin (which zaps our vitality if switched on for long periods of time) and cortisol (which provokes inflammatory responses and weight gain) don't kick in. When our biochemicals aren't focused on mitigating stress, our immune systems function more effectively. We lead happier, more peaceful, joyful, and resilient lives.

A recent study by tapping leader Dawson Church, Ph.D., and his colleagues seems to indicate that tapping works to ease stress. The study included a random sample of eighty-three people who either received one hour of EFT tapping, one hour of traditional talk therapy, or no treatment at all. The EFT tapping subjects' stress hormone levels dropped an average of 24 percent to 50 percent after just that one hour. They reported a corresponding drop in anxiety, stress, and other emotional symptoms. The other groups experienced no similar change.[15]

What if you used the knowledge about tapping and stress regularly? What if each time you started to feel stress coming on, you stopped and tapped first just like you did at the beginning of this chapter instead of going into combat mode? Imagine that when you got to work, you found a demanding email from a company director and you were able to immediately tap on the upset so that you could respond from your center and from peace? What if one by one, bit by bit, you could neutralize the emotional triggers that stress you out? How would your life feel then?

Exercise: Determining When You Get Stressed Out

Step 1. In your EFT journal, create a section called "Stress Release." Ask yourself, when do you get stressed out? What are the stress areas in your life? Write down your answers. For example: I get stressed out when I have four or more different types of tasks to do in one day on my mind and am unclear about priorities. Thinking about the contractors. Family gatherings. Family obligations. When the kids' carpool driver is late. Driving in traffic. When people don't listen to me. When I look in the mirror. At the gym, when I think

15. Dawson Church, PhD, "The Effect of EFT on Stress Biochemistry."

other people's bodies look so much better than mine. Paying the bills. When I get unexpected bill increases. Watching the news.

Step 2. How could you turn your stressful moments into tapping transformation opportunities? When the stress starts coming on, what if you could catch yourself before becoming overwhelmed? All you need to do is stop and rate how stressful the day feels right now. Note where you feel the stressful day in your body. If you're not sure, guess at a place where you might be holding the stress.

Step 3. Create an EFT setup statement for a tapping round that relates to one of the stresses you listed. Give this stressor a nickname: "the blob," "too much work," "out of control," "crazy kids," or "annoying husband." Where do you feel this stressor in your body?

Create a tapping phrase that incorporates your sensory feelings as well. For example, when Ken thought of stress as he performed this exercise, he thought of the pain on the left side of his neck that comes and goes. When he asked himself what brings this pain on, the first thought that came to mind was: "when my girlfriend gives the kids drinks with red dye in them that she knows are bad for them and that makes them hyperactive."

As he tuned into a specific event when this happened, he felt the stress rising and the pain in his neck substantially intensified—this was his tapping target. After two rounds, his anger released, and his neck pain vanished.

Now it's your turn. Got a tapping target? What's your intensity rating on the 0 to 10 scale? Create an EFT statement and perform the EFT basic recipe. Remember to tap on all aspects that are bothering you one at a time until you feel the stress level subside.

Here are examples:

> ***Karate chop:*** Even though there's too much to do and I feel this tightness in my shoulders, I accept myself and how I feel.

Karate chop: Even though I am already so stressed out and tight all over and it's only 7 am, I'm okay. I deeply and completely accept myself.

Each of these would be a separate tapping round. Eventually, you may be able to identify quite a few specific stressors. Just note their intensity, create tapping setups relating to what your day-to-day stressors are, and set them aside until you have the time and energy to tap on them. Tapping isn't meant to create added stress in your life, but to ease it up. Do you see how tapping on statements like the ones above can loosen the stranglehold stress can have on you?

Step 4. When you tap on stress for just five minutes, your whole outlook can change, which in turn can change your life.

As you continue to deepen your practice, you will be able to uncover the specific events that are the table legs holding up your stress with the goal of collapsing the entire reactive stress tabletop in your life.

Where Stress Patterns Originate

Most stress response patterns are laid down at a very young age. They are unconsciously modeled by our family, not calculatedly splashed across the front pages of the newspaper. From newborn to age seven, we are essentially sponges, absorbing ways of being and patterns of behavior from the central figures in our early lives. So our stress reactions imprint at this time—or even earlier—as we mirror theirs.[16]

Studies show that a developing baby in the womb absorbs what Mom is going through, too. A study of expectant New York City moms who suffered PTSD from the 9/11 tragedy and whose babies were born shortly thereafter showed that their babies exhibited a

16. Mercola.com, "EFT Helps Improve Your Health By Freeing Yourself from Stress," Accessed January 11, 2015, articles.mercola.com/sites/articles/archive/2013/04/25/eft-relieves-stress.aspx.

higher stress distress response than other babies.[17] Other epigenetic studies have revealed that seriously stressful events are passed down to the next generation. For example, those whose ancestors lived through a famine may have inherited body traits that hold onto food, which results in a propensity for obesity or unreasonable attitudes about food; those whose ancestors lived through a Holocaust or massacre may have a lower stress tolerance level.[18]

However, not everything derives from our nature. Nurture is also a component in our lives. As we grow aware of our in-built patterns of distress, we can apply tapping, mindfulness, massage, and other approaches to process them, transform them, and experience relief. Let's take a look at working with pattern origins.

Exercise: Exploring Origins of Stress

Questions to ask about inherited and default patterns of stress:

Step 1. Write "Stress Release" as a new heading in your EFT journal. Answer the following questions. When did the central figures in your early life get stressed? Name some specific times when they or you were stressed. How do you know they were stressed? What happened when they were stressed? How did they handle stress? What did you do when you saw they were stressed? Were certain times of the day, night, or year more stressful than others? What stressful incidents and stories do you remember growing up? What stories did you tell yourself as a result of the stress? Where do you find yourself acting in the same way as your mom or dad

17. The Guardian, "Pregnant 9/11 Survivors Transmitted Trauma to Their Children, September 9, 2011," last modified September 09, 2011, www.theguardian.com/science/neurophilosophy/2011/sep/09/pregnant-911-survivors-transmitted-trauma.

18. Danielle Simmons, PhD, "Epigenetic Influences and Diseases," Scitable by Nature Education, accessed January 11, 2015, www.nature.com/scitable/topicpage/epigenetic-influences-and-disease-895.

without being able to help it? What stress stories were common in your family?

Step 2. Look at your list of early-life stress-stories. The preceding questions have doubtlessly led you to many specific events. Give each one a name and rate its intensity. You may tap on them one at a time, using the techniques that you have learned so far, like Tell the Story and Tearless Trauma. When you tap on each of these stories, you might be surprised at the flood of emotion that comes up for release.

Ancestral Stress

Consider tapping on what I call "ancestral stress." In my case, I might tap on anything that comes to mind about my ancestry, uncensored. In this, don't worry about political correctness, but address any raw, archetypal, fairy-tale-type fears that come to mind. I've personally tapped on thoughts and fears like the following that have come to my mind:

> Even though we've been chased out of many a place....
>
> Even though it's not been safe to settle down for any length of time....
>
> Even though I don't feel safe here....
>
> Even though I have a history laden with fighting and jealous ancestors....
>
> Even though the Holocaust happened and I get upset each time I think about it....
>
> Even though we've been playing out this issue for centuries....

Stress Patterns That Show Up as We Grow Older

When we are in our teens and twenties, we have more "give" in our bodies—more health, vitality, and flexibility to survive in the face of stressful experiences. However, as long as we have unresolved stressful experiences from childhood, we are still experiencing unconscious default stress patterns. That would be just fine, except that we don't stay young forever.

Our unconscious stress response patterns build up as we age. At some point, the bucket gets full and then the stress can affect our emotional health and our physical health. You've surely heard things such as: "After the (bad event), my anxiety got really bad." Or, "After Mom died, I started having the pain and went on disability." In most cases, the problem didn't start just then; it had probably been building for years. It's probably been a pattern all of our lives, only now we have the opportunity to deal with things differently.

When a big event comes along, the bucket spills over immediately and the secret is revealed: your stress response is so big that your body can no longer keep a lid on it. Your body is just doing what it has always done, however—listening to your thoughts, feelings, and beliefs about something and then reacting with a biological stress response. That's how seemingly "just one" stressful event can lead to significant trauma.

You begin to ask yourself when the first time you felt stress like this was. When's the first time you had a feeling in your body that feels like this? What does today's feeling remind you of from earlier years? Use your body as a guide, pay attention to the sensations that arise, and tap on them. These often lead a person to a specific early childhood event where the stress reaction pattern originated or the cause of the current-day problem.

Traumatic Stress with a Capital T

Sometimes, just one big trauma has set a stress pattern in motion. Jan Luther, EFT founding master, talks about this pivotal time as the moment everything changed—when a person is seriously injured in a crash, an assault, when a loved one is murdered, and so on.[19] When you are working through traumatic stress, it can be especially helpful to work with an experienced EFT practitioner.

Belief Systems and Stress

Until my body's breakdown forced me to get off that hamster's wheel, nothing was going to change. Looking back, I can now see that enforced rest was the best thing that could have happened. The body never lies. I began listening to my body and partnering with it. I realized that restoring it was the most productive, loving thing I could do—for me and my family. It was a giant step, understanding that the first loyalty I had was to take care of myself. I am a single mama and the hub of the wheel; more than one person depends on me being healthy.

As soon as I slowed down enough to actually feel what was going on in my body and include my body in the process, I became peaceful rather than terrified. I didn't deny my feelings—I leaned into them and embraced them. I tapped on them along with my judgments and my inner voices. I said no a lot more, including to myself, and set boundaries around my time. Finally, I understood my belief until then was that answers to my problems were outside of me. It turned out that I had the answers all along, right in my body.

When that top layer of worry, fear, and negative talk was lifted and those big belief freighters began to turn around, it became clear that the more rest I got, the less upset I became, the better I felt, and the better I was to my son and those around me. My stresses didn't change, I did. My relationship to stressful situations transformed with

---

19. Jan Luther, Email Newsletter and podcast talks, www.janluther.com.

me. Work got easier, faster, more effective, more efficient, and more creative. I was exercising a different muscle than the default stress response; I was strengthening the muscle of trust, compassion, and love for myself, somehow all thanks to a total stress response body burnout. So in fact, stress is a really useful tool, and the sooner you listen to it the less difficult the wake-up call will be.

We don't need to fall apart, get dramatic, or get sick when things get difficult. Truly, tapping offers a way for us to schedule our temper tantrums and nervous breakdowns! Tapping can help us determine what is really true, what is really necessary, and what thoughts, behaviors, and beliefs are actually driving more stress our way. Then we can make better decisions, moving toward a healthier and more effective stress responses.

"I Can't Take a Break" Stress

Stressed-out people believe they can't take a break or things will fall apart, even as they know they are living impossible lives. When you feel like it's impossible to stop, that's the most appropriate time to slow down and rest. Belief systems that harm us seem real, but they are not true. For example, does your family have a belief system that it's not okay to nap or take time off or just do something for fun? You might want to work on that one.

Exercise: "I Have Too Much to Do" Belief System

If you believe you have too much to do and can't take a break (or you can't take the time to exercise even though you love it), try this exercise to transcend the limiting belief. This exercise is in two parts.

Part 1: Decreasing the Intensity

Step 1. What happens when you consider doing something for yourself in the middle of your busy day? Something that will help calm you down, possibly even experience a joy, whether that's taking five minutes to simply slow down and breathe or take a nap? Look at that statement again: "I have too much to do and I can't take a break."

Step 2. How true does it feel that you have too much to do and can't take a break? Let's say that 10 is absolutely true, while 0 is not true at all for you.

Step 3. Take a moment to experience the sensations in your body relating to "I have too much to do and can't take a break." Note in your EFT journal *where* you are feeling any body awareness or sensations about this "too much to do" belief.

Step 4. For this exercise, you are going to tap on the most intense feeling relating to having too much to do. Here's an example of a global EFT setup statement you can customize. "Even though I have too much to do and can't take a break (or whatever other phrase comes to mind), I deeply and completely accept myself."

Step 5. Tap the EFT sequence of points once or several times, starting with the top of the head, customizing this reminder phrase: "Too much to do, I can't take a break." Tap until you experience a shift in intensity.

Step 6. What came to mind as you tapped? Anything specific about your too much to do belief? Jot down any specific events that came to mind about your setup phrases such as one person's response: "If I don't get to these things today, I'll forget, and important things won't get done." You'll use these phrases later to tap on your own and see what's underneath the concerns. Say the statement again to test your progress: "I have too much to do. I can't take a break." Does it feel as true to you? Are you having as many feelings about the "too much to do" belief? Have the feelings changed?

....

When tapping on a belief like this, you might begin to experience the belief as less true or insistent. Perhaps you now feel like it's not necessarily true *all* the time; you may realize there are times during your day that you can—and do—take breaks, for example. Perhaps after a tapping round like this you might suddenly feel the weight of "too much to do" in your body and feel very tired. Or maybe you are feeling sorry for yourself, angry at the world, or resentful of others. Each of these feelings or thoughts is another tapping round. Tap on whatever thoughts come up.

Before we move to the next step, what happened in your body as you tapped? Are you still feeling the same body sensations as when you said "I have too much to do?" Notice that it's common for your body to work along with you, too. You may be experiencing a whole host of sensations as you tap on "too much to do," ranging from numbness to tightness in the chest, a feeling of sheer exhaustion to nausea. Note every physical sensation in your EFT journal, because it means your body is working with you, helping you understand how stress affects it. Can you see how many big feelings you are sitting on that are playing a role in how you are experiencing stress and the decisions you are making? Decreasing the intensity around the "truth" of our beliefs loosens up the stress factor in your body, and that's a good start.

Part 2: Too Much to Do—Getting More Specific

What feeling arises when you think about "I can't take a break. I have too much to do"? Go ahead and input whatever the feeling is into your setup statement. Here's an example of what I mean: "Even though important things won't get done if I take a break and I feel panic when thinking about everything I have to do, I deeply and completely accept myself." Or: "Even though I have too much to do to take a break and that's sad, I deeply and completely accept myself." We'll use the example of "sad that I have too much to do."

Step 1. Rate the sadness or your own feeling about having too much to do on the 0 to 10 scale.

Step 2. Customize this example to target your own specific emotion around "too much to do," repeating the statement one to three times while karate chopping: "Even though I have too much to do, and that makes me feel sad, I love, honor, and accept myself anyway."

Step 3. Tap the EFT sequence once or more using your reminder phrase: "I'm feeling (your emotion) that I can't take a break because I have too much to do."

Step 4. Recheck your intensity. If you are feeling relief, then ask yourself again why you can't take a break, and no doubt another aspect will appear. For example, maybe you can't take a break because you don't know how to stop. Tap on that.

If the intensity is the same or higher, it's time to get more specific. Let's get more specific about times you felt sad because of too much to do. Write your answers down. For example, "I had to miss my son's birthday party," "feeling like my spouse and I are strangers at our anniversary dinner," "when I was running to catch the train and felt like I was going to collapse." You can select one part of any of the above situations and turn it into a specific event of three minutes or less to tap on. For example, "I had to miss my son's birthday party," a couple specific events might be: "The sinking feeling in my stomach when I realized I wouldn't make it to the party on time," and "The closed, unhappy look on my son's face when I came home and they were cleaning up."

File these important specifics under the Stress Relief section of your EFT journal for tapping when you are ready and have the time and energy. You can always take your work with you to an EFT practitioner, too. And as you tap on these, they may likely lead you to the core causes of "can't take a break, too much to do."

While this next bit isn't part of the exercise, it's an alternative to traditional EFT. You will see that I vary the EFT tapping setup statements.

See if any of these ring true for you. If so, test your intensity and perform an EFT round on one or more of them.

> Even though I have too much to do, and that makes me feel (angry, sad, resentful, hopeless, anxious, panicky, all tight, full of despair, or exhausted) and a whole host of other feelings, I would like to experience my life differently.
>
> Even though I have an impossible life with too much to do, but I can't stop because (list what's impossible, such as: too many people are depending on me, important things won't get done…) and I've got big unpleasant feelings inside of me about that, I deeply and completely accept myself and forgive myself for anything that I may be doing to contribute to my impossible life.
>
> Even though I'm exhausted and in despair about having too much to do, I accept all of me and my situation, including the "too much to do" part.

Here's an example of some alternative tapping sequences about "too much to do":

Top of head: I have too much to do and a lot of feelings about that.

Inside eyebrow: I'm sad, exhausted, and feel anger and resentment.

Side of eye: My body feels tight and tired with all this stuff to do.

Under eye: I am feeling really unhappy about having too much to do.

Under nose: It's exhausting to have this much to do all the time.

Chin: I feel (sad, angry, depressed, guilty, unhappy, or full of despair), and a lot of other big feelings about this impossible situation.

Collarbone: It's been this way for a while now, and I'm in despair, because I don't know if I'll ever get the rest I need.

Under arm: It feels impossible, this too-much-to-do situation.

When you tap, you begin to have enough of a cognitive and emotional shift that you might realize there's another way to think about the to-do list. In addition, you might realize you have resources right at your fingertips—but you need to get yourself out of fight-flight and the energy disruption first.

EFT Reframes and Stress

Reframes offer a different way of perceiving the problem, a different perspective. When they land, it's like rain soaking into dry earth, watering all the seeds so they can come to life above ground. We often use reframes but don't consciously know what they are. You might want to take inspiration from the following reframe—another way to look at your stress. Please note, however, that according to many practitioners and official EFT, reframes are not meant to be used unless and until you have cleared enough of the negative intensity from the tapping target. At that point, here's what a reframe might look like:

> Even though I believe I need to control things, what if I could relax and let go? What if I don't have to figure everything out?
>
> Even though it feels like I can't let go, I'm open to the possibility that relaxing might open more doors for me.
>
> Even though I have to hold on tight to the reins because otherwise everything will fall apart, what if it were possible to loosen my grip and relax?
>
> Even though I have to solve all my problems all by myself, I'm open to seeing this differently today/getting help from unexpected quarters.

When a reframe doesn't land, you will hear the resistance loud and clear. You might even get angry about it. Both are also opportunities to tap on the issues the reframe brings up.

Exercise: The "Should" Belief System (BS) and Stress

How does it feel when you hear yourself saying things like, "I should get this done," "I should have done that," "I shouldn't be doing this?" Now consider: "I choose to get this done," "I would rather have done that," "I would prefer to let go of/release/allow/open…" Which feels better?

Are you "shoulding" all over yourself? What are your "shoulds" and "should-nots"? List the "shoulds" and "should-nots" you carry along with you in your journal. Use them as clues to uncover events driving your stress. Let's take an example of the person who as soon as he starts to relax and enjoy himself, says: "I should be doing something productive. I shouldn't be enjoying myself. I have so much to do!" The next questions would be: "What's fearful about enjoying myself?" The answer might be: "In my family, being productive was valued." "What's the downside about relaxing?" Answer: "It's being lazy, which is bad."

The man would get even more specific by asking: "How do I know that being productive was valued while relaxing was equated with being lazy?" The answer likely uncovers a boatload of specific events to tap on here, and this is how you chunk down global issues or tabletops (such as stress) into bite-sized, specific events or table legs. As you know by now, tap on enough of them and you collapse the entire unhealthy stress response, just by looking at the word "should."

Along with "should," phrases and words like "have to," "can't," "never," and "always" don't give us much of a choice about our lives, do they? How does it feel to say "I have to" versus "I choose to," for example? Look at where these words show up in your life and switch the word with a more encouraging phrase, such as "choose," "prefer," "often," "open to trying," "will consider," etc.

In Conclusion

As you aim EFT at the foundational table legs holding up your tabletop of stress, you will find yourself better able to experience stress in a responsive, balanced manner. In turn, this will ease the stress and open up new avenues of thinking, being, and experiencing your life. It may even head off a depression, because you'll begin to feel more hopeful about your life.

In the next chapter, we explore tapping on physical aches and pains, sudden injuries, and serious illness.

Chapter 8

Tapping on the Physical—Illness, Injury, Pain & More

Here you'll explore how to connect with your body no matter the state so you can experience the connection as a resource for healing and well-being. We'll look at the tapping for the Chase the Pain technique, applying tapping in cases of sudden injury, pain, and serious illness, sick children, and to boost immune system resilience.

Like the chameleon that changes color according to the temperature and surface she lands on, so too do our bodies shift and change according to our moods. Our bodies are more responsive than we can possibly imagine. How, really, does a wound heal, a backache go away, or a broken bone knit itself back together? How often do you slow down enough to feel how your leg actually takes just one step, or to truly follow all the adjustments your body makes for you to reach your arm over your head? The way our bodies work (indeed, just pondering the body itself) is deeply mysterious, even unfathomably remarkable.

Have you heard of the Slow Food movement? It was started by Carlo Petrini in 1986 as an effort to combat fast food, encouraging the use of local and cuisine, fresh produce, and sustainable farming. There are also plain slow (body) movements like the Feldenkrais

Method, Body-Mind Centering, the Anat Baniel Method, qi gong, and tai chi. When we slow down enough to feel our bodies with acceptance, we can begin to heal. However, we often disregard the body's needs, or downright abuse it. And yet our body is our partner in life, inevitably intertwined with who we are.

If your body was in charge and you were the silent partner, would you want it to treat you the way you treat it, feel, think, and talk about it? For those of us who have experienced chronic pain, lived with a long-term illness, or have otherwise been challenged by "life in a body," as a friend puts it, we often have some intensity thinking about our bodies. If you are feeling some intensity as you read this right now, how about tapping on those feelings?

Exercise: Intensity about My Body: Global Tapping

Step 1. Write "Tapping on the Physical" as your topic in your EFT journal. Ask yourself if there's something about your body that you don't like. Is it about the way you look or about a certain part of your body that's "giving your trouble"? Is it about weight issues? Is it about illness or pain? Are you feeling sad about how you treat your body? Are you angry/resentful/disappointed at your body for letting you down? Are you frustrated because you can't seem to get your body to do what you want it to do? Are you scared because you can't get better right away? Are you worried about anything that might happen in the future? If nothing comes up to tap on, you can skip this exercise or tap surrogate for somebody else who is sick or having difficulty with his or her body. Remember, surrogate means that you tap "as if" you were someone else. Choose one issue from the list you have created. This will be your tapping target.

Step 2. On the 1 to 10 scale, rate your intensity. For an example, we will start with a global phrase such as: "I am frustrated with my body because it's not doing what I want it to do." Select your own tapping target based on what you wrote in step 1. Or you can follow along with the example. Let's say that I'm at a 7 on the intensity scale regarding frustration with my body because it won't do what I want it do to.

Step 3. Start the EFT setup part of the basic recipe. Karate chop while tuned into the intensity: "Even though I am frustrated with my body because it's not doing what I want it to do, (or insert your own setup phrase), I deeply and completely love, honor, forgive, and accept myself."

Alternative positive affirmations I have used in the past include:

> Even though I'm frustrated with my body because it won't do what I want it to do, *I would like to feel okay about it.*

> Even though I'm frustrated with my body because it won't do what I want it to do, *I wonder if there will ever come a day when I can think of my body and its situation with neutrality.*

You would use these affirmations if they feel right or true to you. Otherwise, just use the basic affirmation: "deeply and completely accept myself."

Step 4. Perform the EFT sequence using the same reminder phrase throughout, starting with the top of the head through under the arm. Here's our example: "frustrated with my body because it won't do what I want it to do." You might tap through several sequences as you hold the feeling in mind until you sense a shift in intensity.

Step 5. What is the intensity surrounding your tapping target now? If it has gone down to zero, has something else come to mind that is more specific about your tapping target? For example, with "frustrated with my body," maybe the person, Chris, is frustrated because his knees have been bothering him for about six months now and they haven't gotten any better. The problem with his body is preventing him from playing basketball, running, and biking, the main ways he used to socialize, relax, and exercise. He can choose to tackle the next aspect, such as "no matter what I do, they don't get better," or "I really miss being active," and so on.

A key question for physical ailments is: What was going on in your life just before or after the issue you're experiencing now? When Chris asks that question, he remembers it's about the time his "difficult" and elderly father who lives across the country got very sick. Chris was conflicted about staying with him and taking time off work to care for and love him or steering clear and doing what he's done most of his adult life—staying away and feeling guilty. He aims EFT at "the conflict," a few specific and troubling events during the time, and how he wanted it to be different but couldn't change how he felt about his dad. As he taps on these issues and some key early "Dad-bad" memories, his knees lighten up, he begins exercising again, and his feelings about his father completely transform to love and forgiveness.

What's underneath your intensity about your body issue? Ask yourself questions again: What is your body "preventing" you from doing? When is the first time you felt this way about your body? What have you tried that didn't work? What was happening in your life around the time things changed or you became aware of the unhappiness with your body? Any of these questions will likely elicit some specific events relating to your emotion surrounding your body. And remmeber, just tracking symptoms also brings relief.

Step 6. Did a specific event come to mind? By answering the previous questions, you likely have a few specific events in mind relating to "frustrated with my body," or whatever tapping phrase you chose to work on, so choose one. Is the event under two or three minutes in length? Give it a title as if it were a scene in a movie, then tap on the event using Gold Standard EFT, tapping all aspects down to zero until that one event no longer bothers you. Now, drop your awareness into your body and ask yourself how your body feels right now.

As we continue, you can choose to tap and read, by continuously tapping on one or more of the tapping points or tapping on the finger points (see the figure in appendix A to locate them if you're not sure.)

The Body and Love

We take our physicality for granted and don't typically consider what an exquisite instrument our body really is. We conveniently manage to forget that we need our body to live. For many of us, it's only when we suffer a problem with our body such as a scratchy throat, serious illness, acute injury, or chronic pain, or when difficult emotions or stress tighten our muscles, that we begin to pay more attention, and that attention is mostly *negative*. We want to get better right now! We get mad at our bodies: "Hurry up and heal already!" "My body has let me down." We talk about our bad leg, problem shoulder, or how we must get rid of the pain right away. Is it any wonder that addiction to painkillers is on the rise? Emotional pain is also something we tend to avoid. One in ten Americans now take an antidepressant, and one in four women in their forties and fifties are on antidepressants.[20]

But what if some types of emotional and physical pain are stemming from the same energy disruption—remember the zzzt! that happens when we experience an event as traumatic that leads to negative emotions? Big feelings are beneath our conscious mind but alive and well in our subconscious, the larger part of the mind. And those big feelings take a toll on our bodies. What if, for example, the pain is emotional that has been stored in the body and is now physically

20. Roni Caryn Rabin, "A Glut of Antidepressants," New York Times Online, Last modified August 12, 2013, well.blogs.nytimes.com/2013/08/12/a-glut-of-antidepressants/?_r=0.

manifesting as well? What if we asked ourselves, regarding a sore throat, for example, questions like these: "What is it that I can't seem to express that hurts my throat," or "What is that lump in my throat saying," or "What are these emotions that are so painful in my throat?"

When we demand healing and dislike our bodies, it's like erecting a dam in the exact place where you want healing to flow like water. We are slowing down the healing process and blocking our path back to health and well-being.

By now you know that our bodies are repositories for our emotions. Along with our external experience, what we think, say, believe, and feel, affect our physical well-being. Our body chemistry is continually shifting and adjusting according to what we are thinking, feeling, saying, believing, and experiencing. When we feel good, we are emotionally connected and in a state of healing; this is the case even when we're sick, injured, and even when we are dying.

It comes as no surprise that "presence," both emotional and physical, is good for us. Presence increases the level of an enzyme in our body called telomerase. This substance both repairs and maintains the ends of our chromosomes, which facilitates health and longevity.[21] Tapping helps access presence—that elusive state of which Buddhists speak.

In reading and exploring EFT, how has tapping affected your body so far? What have you noticed physically during and after tapping? Reports of feeling lighter, more energized, more optimistic, increased vitality, and better sleeping are common. After people experience neutrality or a cognitive shift through tapping, they may notice a feeling of calm, expansiveness, or lightness in their bodies. If they have not felt their emotional or sensory feelings around a "big" issue and are only now tapping into the intensity of it, they might feel re-

21. Dan Siegel, *Brainstorm: The Power and Purpose of the Teenage Brain*, 2013, (New York: Jeremy P. Tarcher/Penguin, 2013), 113.

ally sleepy or shaky after a session. Occasionally when a client reports feeling trembly or shaky during a session, I suggest we shake a bit before we continue tapping. Shaking or vibrating is a natural reflex that releases muscle tension and calms the nervous system. Trauma Release Exercise (TRE) is all about shaking to prevent trauma.

When in the midst of a big upset, many people report feeling awful, experiencing spiking unbearable pain, nausea, fatigue, shakiness, heaviness, numbness, or other interesting feelings as they tap. These troubled sensations and feelings all pass quickly.

Since the body and mind are intimately connected, we can focus on the physical sensations a person is feeling relating to an emotional issue or troubling event. This relationship is of great benefit, especially for those who have "big" emotions about an event or situation. It is possible to focus entirely on a person's physical symptoms to collapse a deeply troubling emotional event while not getting lost in the depths of the emotion. You can consider physical aspects just as you would emotional aspects—individual components that are holding a specific incident in the energy disturbance. The technique you will learn now is called Chasing the Pain.

Introduction to Chase the Pain

Still having a hard time believing that pain can jump around in your body and that it is tied to a feeling you are experiencing? Still believe it's all in your head? Well, in a sense, it is. The state of your mind often affects the state of your body. For example, a client whose leg was amputated at the thigh some two-plus decades prior suffered phantom limb pain for nineteen years—until she tried EFT. In my own EFT practice of fifteen years, I have never come across someone who had worse pain. Her pain on a good day was about a 9 in intensity. She typically described it as if someone were taking pliers and trying to pull off her toe (that wasn't there).

At age 74, Arianna was unable to function without taking pain meds, requiring up to six a day, the maximum, and it had some unpleasant side effects. I don't think I have ever come across a more convenient storage space for undigested traumatic experiences and emotions than a leg that isn't present in the way that most of us would agree a leg is present. As we worked, tapping on the specific painful memories/events using Tell the Story, one at a time inside what we called her "unleg," her pain resolved to the point that she no longer needed pain medication.

Now, when pain does arise, she does her pacing, which means she taps as she wheelchairs from room to room until the pain subsides. Arianna has also resumed activities such as going to church, taking daylong outings, writing books, and more.

What happens most times is when a person taps on one specific event, the pain in their bodies jumps all over the place during the unraveling of the story's intensity, dissipating with the resolution of the energy disruption.

In Arianna's case, her pain would jump all around her foot and leg that weren't there. So, if we were tapping Tell the Story on a specific event, such as "When I got the phone call from the hospital about Danny," or the "Wild West Fiasco," the unbearable pincer pain might start at the toe and then expand to all the toes, then it would change to a burning sensation, then it might feel like her whole foot was being sawed off at the ankle, then it would shift again to a scratchy feeling, and then it would disappear completely—in exact accordance to her complete neutrality around our tapping target.

While Arianna was feeling this pain, I wasn't insensitive to her anguish, but I also knew that the pain was relating to the part of the story that she was on in Tell the Story. I was merely tracking her pain as we kept the primary focus on the story's emotional aspects she was unraveling with Tell the Story. It was pretty profound.

Please note, I managed these sessions extremely closely so she didn't get lost in any messes after the sessions. She also had mental health support and other resources in addition to working with me. As we had rapport and a longer-term clinical relationship, I knew how much she could handle. This is important especially when working with severe trauma, as she had experienced. If you find yourself falling deeper into a hole and tapping isn't helping, it means you need additional resources, such as a mental health expert and an experienced EFT professional. I have also worked in conjunction with mental health professionals per legal permission of the client.

Gold Standard EFT Technique: Chasing the Pain

Chasing the Pain is the physical counterpart to the Tell the Story and Movie techniques covered in chapter 4. This time, however, the story is not one you tell with your words—it's the one your body is generously sharing with you as the pain or awareness shifts throughout it while you tap. For example, perhaps the emotional upset relating to something that happened between you and your partner this morning is a 10 on the rating scale. In your body, you feel tightness in your shoulders as you think of the words that were said. Instead of going into the story about the argument, start tapping on the body sensation, creating an EFT setup that reflects the tight shoulder feeling. The pain often shifts, as the technique's name implies. Maybe now the awareness of pain might shift to your heart, which feels heavy. You would then tap on the heavy heart feeling. Then the pain might jump back to the shoulders but perhaps a little bit down to the right. The pain can literally jump around like a ping-pong ball in a high-stakes game. Your job is to track the pain and tap on it as it moves around until finally you experience relief from both pain and the starting emotional upset. As the physical pain lessens, the tapper also experiences an emotional release.

If you don't have a specific incident relating to your body concern, no matter. You don't even need to know the specific incident upon which you are tapping because your body knows and is doing the work on your behalf. You can feel your way through the story with your body as guide.

Chase the Pain also allows you to sneak up, if you will, on an emotional issue by tapping on the symptoms in the body relating to the issue. It spares the user excess emotional pain by focusing on physical symptoms instead. The conscious mind gets so caught up in tracking the physical, that the normal walls a person would put up in going to a painful emotional place are bypassed altogether. Sneaky, and it works—quickly.

The Chase the Pain technique often links a body sensation to a specific, emotionally charged incident and then releases both the pain and charge of the event; oftentimes the body sensations will do it for you. Sometimes, you will need to tap on the emotional aspects relating to the event.

Is knowing what the incident was to resolve the physical symptom essential? No. For example, many of us experienced birth trauma—fetal distress syndrome, premature labor, a C-section, induced birth, suction birth—when we were born, and the ensuing fear of being stuck in the birth canal or separated from mother post-birth. We have no conscious memory of that or what any ensuing emotions are linked to, yet the sensory feelings and emotions are still there. We can tap on the body feeling; we don't need to be conscious of the content. It's okay to tap on feelings that arise.

With Chase the Pain, we are not trying to get rid of pain or symptoms; rather we are softening into them. We are nonresistant, going into the feeling of the symptoms fully and deeply with our full attention while tapping, in full acceptance with an affirmation. We simply chase the pain around the body, a process that often leads to core issues still held in the body's tissues that in my practice leads to regular relief from physical symptoms. Addressing the physical can resolve the emotional. Addressing the emotional can resolve the physical. They are interwoven by design. After all, it's within the body where feelings first arise.

This synergistic combination is powerful enough that it can in many cases bring relief to numerous body symptoms, unraveling the incidents and emotions underlying the physical pain altogether. Please note that I'm not stating a direct correlation between illness and emotion or in any way saying that we cause our own illness. Life is far more complicated than this type of black-and-white thinking. What I am saying is that tapping can help manage pain and calm you down.

A colleague who had been sidelined with back pain for decades used Chase the Pain and would often get good results, but certain circumstances when she wasn't supported would bring all the symptoms back quickly. Her breakthrough in back pain relief came when she had a realization: "I didn't need to tap on other people's anger. Rather, I needed to acknowledge their anger and then tap on all the reasons, images, words, and feelings around my own anger."

Case Study: Relief from "Love Hurts" Belief with Chase the Pain Technique

Lois, age 41, is an entrepreneur and serious amateur athlete. Unfortunately, she had been sidelined for the past several months by severe, mysterious (according to the doctors), fibromyalgia-like pain.

She sought me out for pain relief: "It hurts so much," she said. Years back, Lois had let go of the idea of marriage, so when she met a wonderful man and they decided to marry, she wanted to relish every part of the process, including planning the wedding. He even had three children, of whom he shared physical custody, which fulfilled Lois's dream of having children. However, her horrible pain was marring everything.

The physical pain had started about the time she began planning the wedding. It was so severe it forced her to cut back on her client load and interfered with the joy she had anticipated planning every detail of the wedding.

Lois and I worked together for about four sessions, using Chase the Pain on her worry that she would not get to enjoy her new life. When we first spoke over the phone, she referenced her mother several times, who had tried to control Lois as a child. She had forced her to dress a certain way to keep up appearances, and now she was trying to butt into the wedding plans. Lois was having none of it; this wedding was going to be done *her* way. I heard in Lois's voice the extreme anger about her mother; a clue.

What she shared along with my intuition led me to consider that she was experiencing "mother stuff," and I wondered if it was playing a role in the pain problem. However, Lois didn't want to work on any early memory involving her mother when I asked. "I've done so much mother work," she said, "I'm not willing to do any more." I let it be for the time being. Besides, she was too angry about her today troubles destroying her dreams and life.

We instead employed the Chase the Pain technique on her pain, her upset over being so sick, and her worries about not enjoying her new life. She had been getting worse as the months passed and the wedding drew near.

As we tracked her body pain all over the map, she grew increasingly angry. "It still hurts! Nothing's going to work!" The pain was like a jumping bean, moving from her back to her sacrum to her chest to somewhere else. Each shift was another aspect and tapping round with the EFT basic recipe.

At the end of the session, she started sobbing. A huge emotional dam seemed to have burst, and with it came some emotional and physical relief. In the next session she was ready to tap on a few memories and core issues that had surfaced earlier in her life. The first incident was when she was seven years old: a beloved older sibling turned her away; the second involved a conflict with "keeping up appearances" and big anger in the home. She understood from these traumatic events that "love hurts" and "love isn't safe," beliefs she had evidence for and had lived for the last three decades of her life. In our session Lois released a great deal of grief and the pain significantly subsided.

Our next task was to begin reframing her belief system. We tapped on her helplessness at the time; that her mother didn't know any better and was just doing the best she could. We tapped on the fact that her fiancé was not her mother, and that she could truly have happiness; her body didn't need to protect her from love any more, and she was safe to love. We tested for aspects, running through events slowly and with exaggeration, to see if there were any remaining upset bits that needed to be rooted out. We tapped on the good things that had happened and that were going to happen. Her symptoms disappeared. Last I heard, her wedding took place a few months later, and it was fabulous. Today she is enjoying her new life, pain free.

Exercise: Practicing Chase the Pain

Step 1. Get out your Personal Peace Procedure tapping target list. Which, if any, upsetting event jumps out right now? That's the one you'll use to experience Chase the Pain. Or maybe you have a more pressing issue that has arisen that is not on your list. Use that. You only need to identify something that's bothering you right now.

Step 2. Rate the emotional intensity of your tapping target on the 0 to 10 scale, write down the number, and set it aside. We will start now with Chase the Pain.

Step 3. Review the targeted event in your mind as you would with Tell the Story. Ask yourself: "Where in my body is there a physical sensation that's bothering me?" or "Where in my body is the physical awareness of this upset (from your tapping target) in my mind?" Scan your body for any sensations such as: tightness in your jaw, shallow breathing, a quickening of the pulse, nervous fingers, a clenching feeling in the gut, a sharp pain on the left side in the mid-back, nervous twitch, hot flash, shoulder pain, feeling suddenly tired.

Step 4. Get very focused and curious about the physical sensation without trying to make it go away. Ask yourself: Where is it? How big is it? What shape is it? What's its density? How painful is it? What kind of pain is it—heavy, tight, sharp, dull, achy? You can get really specific; there are no "wrong" answers. Questions that may help: If the pain had a texture, what would it be—cement, silly putty, cookie dough, or water? If my pain had a color, what color would it be? and so on. If you are only aware that you are feeling something in your body that feels off, start there.

Step 5. Now rate the sensation you are having on the 0 to 10 intensity scale. This feedback is critically important when you're performing Chase the Pain, as symptoms will indeed move around and change in intensity.

Step 6. Apply the EFT basic recipe to one specific symptom. You may be having many symptoms, but choose one at a time for best results. If possible, tap it down to zero before moving on to another symptom. Let's say you feel some tightness in your chest when you think about getting your project in before the deadline, or you feel tightness in your chest thinking about having that talk with your spouse or your teenager. As with most examples, keep it simple and don't use heavy or deep issues at this point. Let's look at an example of the setup phrase and EFT sequence we could use for "the tight chest feeling about the talk with teenager or spouse."

Repeat the EFT setup phrase while tapping on the Karate Chop point: "Even though I have this tightness in my chest on the left side about the size of an orange radiating out in a circle, I deeply and completely accept all of me."

Step 7. Tap down the points starting with the top of the head and ending up under the arm. Use a brief reminder phrase such as "my tight chest" or "this tight feeling in my mid-left side" or "this stretched orange tight feeling right behind my heart." Customize your phrase to suit how it feels for you. Tap through the EFT sequence a few times or more, starting with the top of the head point through the inside of the eye point.

As you tap, note any changes in sensation, including spikes or sudden drops in tightness or pain, or if no change occurs.

Step 8. Continue tapping on that one symptom until the sensation shifts or resolves altogether. If you have shifted in your symptom sensation or the symptom has gone away, test based on your original physical description to make sure. If it's a 0 and you have no physical discomfort, then it's time to go back to your specific event, and continue the story until you experience a shift to another pain symptom. Rate your intensity and track that physical symptom. Continue tracking the pain and tapping on each area that arises, tapping down to zero. Once you have resolved each symptom, return to the issue or emotional incident in question and see if the intensity has changed. Often you'll find the incident that bothered you is now down to a zero without you having tapped directly on it at all. Only do one symptom at a time. Manage this carefully. You can't focus on everything all at once.

An easier entrée into tapping on the physical can be to simply track your symptoms one at a time and tap down on them one at a time. You might find as if often the case with my clients that their pain is related to a specific event that comes to mind as they tap on the specific symptom. Just go with it.

Sometimes you'll find that an incident or memory comes to mind as you tap on body sensations, and you may experience a sudden emotional release and simultaneous let-up in the pain. In situations like these, you may also experience a spike in pain before it subsides to zero; be patient and persistent.

Tips for Getting Results with Chase the Pain

Focus wholly on a symptom, shutting off your cell phone or any other distraction. Engage your mind. Here are ways to track pain that will help you get tuned in.

- Identify the exact location and size of the symptom, e.g., directly above my belly button, about the size of a plum.

- Describe the pain's quality, e.g., a dull ache, a throb, a sharp stab, a tight feeling, a wrenching sensation, a heavy feeling, a numb feeling, diffuse feeling that spreads out, a feeling of twisting, burning.
- If the symptom had a color, what would it be? For example: red-orange, fuchsia, black, neon, muddy.
- Describe the symptom's texture, e.g., cement, watery, tarry, like Play-Doh.
- How long has the symptom been there? Since the beginning of time? Since last night?
- Give the pain a nickname, e.g., Old Faithful, My Annoyance, the Blob, Road Runner, the Joker.
- What would the symptom say to you if it could talk? For example: "I'm sick of you not paying attention to me," "you can't ignore me!" Would you be willing to have a conversation with the hurting part of your body?
- What happens if you thank that part of your body for holding all that pain?
- What's the feeling or emotion of the symptom? Ex: Sad, angry, frustrated, hopeless, resistant?
- What do you believe to be true about the pain?
- Figuratively speaking, who might it be stuck in that part of your body? Your mother? An ex? Your boss? For example for neck pain: "that pain in the neck" relates to emotions about the boss; shoulder tension relates to "taking care of Dad is such a heavy weight on my shoulders," leading to emotions about Dad; tightness in ribs and mid-back and chest relates to grieving a loss, which relates to emotions about an accident and love loss. Alternatively, what emotions about that particular person are you carrying in your body?
- Reaffirm your unshakable belief in your ability to heal, however that looks and whatever that means. Reaffirm your

belief that it's possible for other people to heal. Here are some affirmations I regularly express: "There is a part of me that believes it's possible to heal." "I believe in healing." "I am healing, and I am healed." "Other people can heal, I can heal, too." "Part of me has an unshakable belief in myself."

If You Don't Feel Any Change in Your Body Symptoms

It can happen that you feel no change when you tap on a symptom. Try the previous questions and see what shakes out. Start asking yourself questions, too: "Am I getting specific enough in my EFT setup?" Get yourself very interested in what your body is doing. A friend of mine said she didn't feel anything in her body, and then a couple seconds later her stomach gurgled—a sensation! That's where she would go next. Or you could focus on the frustration that you're not feeling anything in your body. There's always something to tap on.

Make sure you've watered and fed yourself enough, as dehydration and too little nourishment can make it more difficult to get results. Other environmental issues can also interfere with results, such as high electrical fields in the case of people with sensitive bodies, and allergies. Ask yourself if you are giving yourself the time and space you need to fully focus. Are you worried about something else while tapping? Are you worried about the symptom or focused on needing it to go away right now? In that case, you might want to first tap on what's the most intense, such as "this worry that won't leave my mind." You could also focus on one of the specific worries that you have before tackling the body symptoms. Most importantly, be gently persistent. Remember that pain is your body's alert system and it lets you know that something needs your attention. Moreover, pain is a signal to care for yourself. Slow down enough to care for you. If you are seriously ill or seriously physically depleted, give yourself plenty of time to tap. If you are exhausted and have visited many different doctors and haven't slept well for days (or years), tapping may take a bit longer. The key is to care for yourself with patience as you would a very small child.

Our Pain and Sickness History Sheds Light on Today Symptoms

Exercise: Releasing Trauma from Sickness and Pain—EFT Journal

How do you experience pain and sickness in your body? What are your experiences relating to pain and sickness? Get your EFT journal and write "Getting Sick" on one page and "Feeling Pain" on the other page. As with the last exercise, I encourage you to take some breaks to tap continuously. And then continue writing. I have found this exercise to be emotional, probably because I have experienced many physical ailments in my life, so it's useful to tap on the disruption. Even if you aren't focusing in on a specific incident, you'll be taking the edge off the intensity.

Step 1. Create two topics in your EFT journal: Sickness and Pain.

Step 2. Under "Sickness," list illnesses you've had that come to mind as well as ones you remember family members having, going all the way back to when you were born. List illnesses you don't remember having but were later told about. These may include: getting a shot at the doctor's, in the hospital waking up after my tonsils were taken out, my brothers told me I always got sick at big events, calling for Mom with a sore throat, throwing up in the teacher's lap at school, learning I had IBS, the cancer scare....

Step 3. Under "Feeling Pain," list times you were in serious pain, witnessed serious pain, any pain you are feeling in your body now, and the first time you recall being aware of something painful. Anything that comes to mind is appropriate to tap on, even if there's no charge. As I've said before, because your subconscious brought it to awareness, there's likely some gold there.

Step 4. Now title each event you listed and note any intensity in the margin.

Step 5. Looking at sicknesses you've had over the years, choose one event from the list with the most intensity, right now. Employ the EFT basic recipe as well as Chasing the Pain (if relevant) until the event intensity subsides to zero, making sure to test your intensity before and after tapping each round.

Step 5a. Administer some self-care. If you are feeling overwhelmed and have continued tapping but are still not making headway, it might be time to pause and allow yourself an emotional rest. Figuratively gather up the event you were tapping on and place it in a box, room, or a place where you don't have to work with it right now. Set it aside.

Step 6. Move on to the next event after the current one has tapped down to neutrality. Tap through each item one at a time using your Personal Peace Procedure approach. (See chapter 4 if you're uncertain about the Personal Peace Procedure.)

Here's an example: Jenny was hospitalized at age six and nearly died. Within the hospitalization experience, she has many different events/memories to tap on, including: *being so hot; held in sister's arms; Mom taking me in the wagon; Mom with me at the bed; the nurse making me eat bad food; not able to talk; getting a present from my aunt; waiting for my mother to come; feeling scared, weak, and lonely.* As she taps, more comes up: *Mom said they couldn't bring the fever down, said I was burning up; Mom said she put me in a cold bath but it didn't help; Mom gave me attention and tea.* Each one of these is a specific incident. Do you see that you can remember more than you think?

Jenny can tap on each of these specific incidents and any and all aspects (components) that arise, including the words her sister and her mother said. She will likely feel a surprising amount of emotion from this old memory and have new insights about her aversion to hospitals and doctors, and her out-of-proportion worry about dying whenever she gets sick. She also realizes this is a core contributor to "I have to get sick to get what I want." After she taps, she'll find her emotions about hospitals and her enmity toward doctors has changed, and she no longer feels the need to make herself weak and no longer gets sick when she is going after something she wants. If she starts to head down that road, she recognizes that she's just having another aspect, and taps on it.

What happens to you emotionally when you get sick or experience pain? It's useful to apply tapping to all the feelings, thoughts, self-talk, and beliefs you can come up with around sickness and pain. When you learn to tap away these old fears, you can take sickness in stride as part of life, and you will generally recover much faster. Your whole life might change for the better.

Pain and Sickness, Secondary Gain, Belief Systems

Secondary gain, or the "upside" of being sick is a common experience. Ask yourself what's the upside of illness? What's the downside of getting well? What would have to change if you got well? What is it that's useful to you when you are sick that you won't have when you are well? Explore the upside with regard to your illness. Jenny had an upside: she got attention and wasn't teased by family members.

In Lois's case, secondary gain nearly sidelined her marriage to the partner of her dreams. In my own case, I came to understand after tapping and healing from my own fibromyalgia that one of my deep-seated subconscious beliefs was that when I was sick, I got love. No one expected anything of me, I wasn't teased, and I got Mom's full attention. Evidently, I understood on some unconscious level "I need to be sick to get love. I need to be sick to be safe."

That's secondary gain—or the upside. It's not conscious but it's operating on the unconscious level. Yikes!

So is it really true that the only time I am lovable is when I am sick? That's a major damper on my life! Obviously that's not true today nor was it back then. This is the problem with our limiting beliefs—they aren't even true, but we just do our level best to make them true for us at the expense of true possibility and joy. From an EFT perspective, my limiting thoughts were associated with the energy disruption I experienced a long time ago based on a core issue around being sick and being hospitalized. I had internalized this belief system as true, even though it wasn't objectively true and had carried this through my entire life. Logically this belief system wasn't true, but it felt true emotionally.

I unraveled the energy disruption relating to this deep-seated belief by looking at the events or table legs that were holding up this tabletop belief system, and tapping on enough of them to collapse the entire tabletop. Even so, once in a while I'll start to feel overwhelmed or feel sick in the "old" way. This is an immediate cue for me to start tapping on another aspect of this belief system. How do I find the aspect? I simply look at what's been going on in my life since I started to feel the sick feeling, and tap. When intensity arises, instead of running around like a chicken with its head cut off (as my grandmother used to say) and falling back into old unhelpful patterns, use these moments to tap and clear out another aspect. Watch for these moments of stress and being overwhelmed for just this reason.

Another issue that used to arise for me was the tension I would start to feel in my neck and shoulders when my schedule for the coming week started to look overly full, even when it was clearly (logically) manageable for me. I'd turn away business and be fearful that it was too much for me in my condition (whatever the particular condition was that week). Is it any wonder that by midweek, I'd feel rundown and sometimes even get sick? I realized that I had a belief system: "If I have what I perceive to be too much on my plate,

I won't be able to handle it, so I should get sick because then I won't have to handle too much." It makes no logical sense, a hallmark of B.S. (belief systems). In fact with clients I'll often ask them to repeat their belief systems slowly and write them down word for word because they make no literal sense. I often repeat what they said back to them, and they begin to realize when hearing their words that what they are saying is not making any sense. That's headway!

Watch for the times when *you* feel overwhelmed or stressed, because these are the moments when you can easily slip into your old default belief systems that don't work for you anymore. If you are having one of these BS moments, don't despair. Try adapting phrases like these:

> Even though I'm doing it again, I shower myself with love and compassion.
>
> Even though my shoulder's starting to go south again, I accept myself and how I feel right now.
>
> Even though I'm scared I'll get sick again if (list the issue here), I deeply and completely accept myself.
>
> Even though I've just stepped into that old hole again, it's getting a lot easier to climb out of, now that I know how.
>
> Even though I've got this belief system that says....
>
> Even though having this experience just triggered me right back into feeling like that helpless, hopeless, scared little girl, I'm remembering that I'm all grown up and am safe and sound.

Each one of the above statements is actually one round of EFT. What would your own EFT setup statements be? Practice writing a few that capture the moment.

The more you use EFT to target your own fears relating to sickness or pain, the more you begin to understand that you are, right now, okay, and that the pain or sickness is *not* all of who you are. This insight may be key for those living with a serious illness or recovering from a serious accident. Sometimes it feels living through a Zen koan, like you need to go on and yet your situation is impossible—tap on that.

Sudden Injury, Accidents, Surgery

Now we'll briefly explore using tapping to resolve pain and trauma from minor cuts to traumatic car crashes or accidents. Although I won't cover assaults in this text, it is common for those who tap on the emotional issues underlying serious traumatic events such as childhood sexual assault, violent crime, or the sudden loss of a loved one, to see many (in some cases, all) physical symptoms, especially pain, clear. These are also the same target population for which the doctors can allegedly do nothing for, in many cases. In my belief system, there is no such thing as a lost cause or a tough case. While tapping doesn't do surgery, it can put you at ease as you are about to go into surgery so your nervous and immune systems aren't on high alert. Tapping can also minimize pain and shorten recovery periods post surgery. EFT can also work on burn relief. Remember the story about the boiling hot water I dropped on my foot in chapter 1? To go a bit more into detail, the boiling wet heat immediately saturated my heel, toes, and left foot, traveling up my ankle. I whimpered to my friend to come help, and as I struggled to get my sock off, the pain seared deep into my foot. I tapped on every aspect I could think of, simply focusing on the sensations and feelings as each arose. Even tapping on the feelings of one with no words works as you are wholly engaged in the topic.

Here are some phrases: "Even though this really really really hurts so bad…," "OHH! OWW!" "I can't believe I did that!" "Ouch, hurts! Ouch, hurts!" "Really, really hurts!"

The pain shifted from off-the-charts to a deeper, burning feeling, and I shifted my focus along with it. When it turned to an ache and a throb, I shifted again, and so on, through each sensation. I tapped on everything that came to mind, including the surprise, the shock, my own disbelief that I had done that, as well as self-talk about how stupid that was and what a loser I was (thanks, inner critic, for helping me return and zap a core limiting belief in my life). The good news, however, is that I kept tapping.

After perhaps ten minutes, the person I was with and I both observed the pain decreasing rapidly with each tapping round. I then provided reassurance to my foot: "The accident is over and we survived. It's okay to go back to normal. You (my foot) are safe and sound. We are safe. You can go back to normal right now. I'm asking my immune system to send healing and soothing to my foot. I'm asking the mucus membranes of the body to soften and coat the area that is inflamed, soothing and cooling the whole area. I want my immune system to know that we don't have to have burns, red marks, and the like; that the pain is over and done with and I'm okay and so is my foot. I'm so grateful for my foot. I'm glad that my foot knows how to heal.

After twenty minutes there was no pain, only two tiny light pink streaks left to tell the tale.

Put EFT in Your First-Aid Kit

After people discover how useful EFT is after physical trauma, it is one of the first items they later pull out of the toolkit in an emergency. If your son has fallen and is bleeding, tap. If your oldest just pulled a hank of hair out of the youngest's head and everyone's wailing, tap. If your elderly mother has just had a fall, tap. If you're afraid that you will fall on the ice outside, tap. If you're being transported to the hospital, tap. If you can't use your hands, imagine tapping inside while tuned in to the fear. If you hear that someone else has been in an accident, tap. If you fear you're going to have a setback and never recover, tap. Just tap on all of the awful ideas that come to mind—so they can release and your immune system can focus on healing instead of on freaking out.

Resolving Trauma of Serious Accidents and Healing

Sometimes, just one significant trauma can wreak havoc in a person's life. For example, in *The Tapping Solution* movie by brother and sister team Nick and Jessica Ortner, I recall a woman featured who had suffered serious injuries in a car crash on a date, and was told she would have some physical disabilities for the rest of her life. In the movie, she tapped with experts on all aspects of the car crash story: what the doctors said, what she didn't like about the date, that the guy was driving too fast, her anger, and more. The results, after tapping on many aspects during the filming? She experienced relief from her emotional trauma and physical issues.

Release Fears and Pain from Past Accidents

In another case, Michael, a professional motocross racer, had two serious accidents within a year. Now his career was at a crossroads. While he had recovered for the most part physically, he was *thinking* his way through his jumps and races, rather than allowing his whole being to flow through at these critical moments. Naturally, he was no longer winning or even placing. His career might soon be over, unless that changed.

We tapped several incidents relating to the accident, from the day getting off to a bad start to the bike not working properly, seeing the turn, landing wrong, being in the hospital, and finally, realizing that he would not race again that year. As we tapped, the various parts of his body that had been injured spoke up and he felt their pain, which then released. Once the trauma and intensity from the issues we tapped on were neutral, he was ready to receive the reframes. We provided reassurance to his body and communicated directly with it, speaking directly to his subconscious, letting his whole being know that it was far safer to actually *not* think his way through the races, but allow the body-mind to flow through the races as it had in the past. After our first tapping round, he placed. After the second tapping, he placed again, and he realized he was no longer thinking his way through the race.

Going Viral: Colds, Viruses, Infections, Allergies, and the Like

Now we'll move on to using EFT to address and provide relief from the pesky viral maladies that plague us with sore throats, runny noses, coughs, fevers, itching, and more.

When you have a symptom or even if you feel that cold coming on that everyone else has and believe there's nothing you can do—tap. Once you resolve the emotions underlying the sore throat or the cough, those will often release. Tap on the scratchy feeling, on the itch, the runny nose, how lousy you feel, not wanting to go to the doctor, the insurance copay, your frustration with your body, the fear that it's going to go into your chest, the difficulty sleeping, why do I keep getting this bug, the kids at my son's school who passed it on, to whatever the symptoms are. Tap on them one at a time and allow the emotion to flow out.

In most cases, you can tap effectively with children, helping them manage their pain and their emotions, too. Here's an example of how EFT worked with my six-year-old neighbor friend, Tasha. I happened to drop by at the time. She was stuck inside on the first day of vacation, while the rest of the kids were all outside playing—she could see them from the window.

I asked young Tasha to describe how her sore throat felt. She said, "It hurts. It's red. And I can't talk," suddenly starting to whisper. I whispered back, and she laughed. It was a good sign; laughter is truly healing balm. When you can laugh, fissures begin to appear in the issue, and it may soon collapse altogether. A recent study has found that laughter puts your brain in the same healing place as meditation, only faster.[22]

---

22. Health Day, "Laughter May Work Like Meditation in the Brain," Study, Last modified April 28, 2014, consumer.healthday.com/alternative-medicine-information-3/mis-alternative-medicine-news-19/laughter-meditation-exp-bio-meeting-llu-release-batch-1149-687061.html.

I will often use my sense of humor in a situation or exaggerate histrionically. If you are ready for this, you will have tapped enough of your upset down and what you say will land, a more advanced EFT technique. We all have a natural sense of humor, but sometimes it gets covered up by hurts.

I asked Tasha: "How big of a hurt is it in your throat? Is it this big?" I opened my arms wide to both sides of my body. "Or this big?" I bent my elbows and brought my arms closer together. "Or this big?" I asked, as I brought the palms of my hands together as if in prayer.

As we talked, I had an intuition that Tasha's illness might be related to her mom, who had started working again. I suddenly realized that today was the first day of school vacation . . . and Mom wasn't there. I kept my observation in mind but didn't say anything yet.

Tasha hadn't been given a say in her mom going back to work, and she was now getting less of her time. Could the feelings about Mom being unavailable be stuck in her throat, contributing to its soreness? I was waiting to see if this would arise as we tapped.

In my client work, I notice that the other person's intuition is often leading them, though they may not be aware of it. For example, when a long-forgotten story from childhood pops into mind as we are tapping on a present-day trauma, I will either bookmark it for later, or suggest that we go there and see what happens, depending on its intensity and their wishes. Generally, these leaps of logic bring us a wealth of results. Perhaps it's intuition or cognition of my experience that when we address earlier issues that are more foundational or core, we often have a bigger collapse of the tabletop issue. Maybe it's your subconscious (after all, it's about 90 percent of your mind) doing what it needs to do to help you heal. It's the limited consciousness of the ego that can truly be irrational. You can begin allowing and trusting that your intuition will become increasingly important as you deepen your EFT work.

Working with little Tasha, we began describing the pain in her own words, "the stingers in my throat feeling." We didn't use the

0 to 10 intensity scale; I knew she wasn't really a numbers person. You don't need to have a number, actually; as noted earlier, there are numerous ways to discern intensity. In this case, I asked her to show me how big it was by opening her arms as wide as it hurt.

Tasha opened her arms wide out to both sides, and then pulled them in a little bit. I guessed it was about an 8. We made up our statement together, and I kept in mind that little children need phrases and words they can relate to: "Even though my throat hurts and it has little stingers in it, I'm an awesome girl and Mom and Dad love me too." I've also used phrases like "Even though (the problem), my dog Ralph loves me," or "... God loves me," or even "my Teddy Bear likes me."

Within five minutes, Tasha's sore throat pain went from arms as wide as she could make them to hands together clasped in prayer position at the heart—that is, no pain at all in the throat. She still felt run down and had a runny nose, but she was laughing. Tapping was entertaining to her. We kept going. A few minutes later, "Mom's not here to be with me," arose as a big wide-armed upset, as I'd expected. We tapped on the sadness that Mom has always been here but now she's not, that Tasha was mad at Mom for not being there, that she believes Mom should be there with her all the time, and more. Not surprisingly, tapping on these feelings caused her stuffy nose and the rundown feeling to disappear as easily as the sore throat. She no longer missed Mom, either. The whole session took maybe fifteen minutes, if that. Soon thereafter, Tasha was outside playing with her friends.

Tapping on Children's Owies, Aches, and Pains

The children I have worked with and those who are tappers on their own rarely need much time tapping to feel better. I sometimes work with props, such as stuffed animals (of theirs or one I have on hand) or puppets. Children can also tap on their parents and it will work. Usually, a child and I tap on the critter as if he or she were experiencing the child's symptoms. For example, in the case of a child suffering from a stomach ache, you might suggest that the little one tap on his or her stuffed critter, saying that Mr. Bear has a tummy ache, and it might help if you tap on these feel-good points. Here are some words to suggest getting the child started: "Even though (this teddy bear) is hurting in his stomach, s/he is a good bear and I love her/him very much."

I'll suggest children tap on Mom or Dad instead of tapping on themselves first if parents are okay with it. Doing so gives the children an added feeling of empowerment. Other times I'll have Mom or Dad tap as if they were the child while the child watches. This also works. Remember surrogate tapping?

Surrogate Tapping Symptoms

You can tap on yourself as if you were your child, even if the child is not in your immediate vicinity. Surrogate tapping works as long as you can stay neutral about your own feelings, and it may take practice tapping to feel really confident about this use of EFT. You might first tap on all the concerns you have about your child's illness, and alternate tapping on your own fears and concerns and your child's symptoms. How do you tap surrogate with a child? Put yourself in their shoes and imagine what they would say if they were tapping.

Going Deeper with Symptoms

Does one part of your body seem to get stricken more often, such as your sinuses, tummy, or throat? Are you tapping as you read? It can help.

When you do get sick, is it always in the same place with the same symptoms? Target that part when you are not sick. Try tapping with EFT setups focused on that part of your body for seven days in a row: your beliefs, thoughts, and experiences of being sick in that way or place. Tap on any incidents that come to mind and you will be tapping on whatever emotions are harbored in those body areas so you won't have to get sick. You are thus creating more resilience in that particular area of your body and life.

Sometimes after a person has had an injury, that area of their body in which they were injured seems to become a repository for chronic pain. Often you will find that emotions from troubling events are housed in that area of your body. In the case of the client with phantom limb pain, it gets even more interesting. Each time she thought of certain specific incidents in her life such as the loss of her partner, the conflict with her former mother-in-law, the difficulties with the doctors who didn't help or listen, the pain in her "unfoot" would increase. She would feel very specific pain that was quite descriptive, and it almost seemed like she was being tortured. As we tapped down on the specific events, the pain cleared.

More on Sickness as Metaphor

Expressions we use every day offer clues: "I have a pain in the neck": Who or what might that be? "It feels like I've been stabbed in the back": When do you feel stabbed in the back? "My hands are tied": When do you feel this way? "It's a real thorn in my side": Who or what do you believe is a thorn in your side? "I'm having a hard time digesting that": What can't you accept? "It feels like the weight of the world is on my shoulders": Who or what are you carrying? Your answers are your own; it's not as though the person is really in or on there. You're investigating your feelings about that person.

A client named Jack had excruciating back pain he described as "a stab in the back." As we tapped on the current-day pain, it came out that he had been betrayed by a fellow weightlifter who had figuratively "stabbed him in the back" by letting the weights he was supposed to be spotting fall on Jack. As we resolved that memory, an even earlier memory of back pain came up that I considered a core issue. Again, core issues are events that play a role in shaping our lives. As it happened, his little brother used to tell on him even when he had done nothing wrong. Jack's father would suddenly slam him on the back in that exact place. Jack was stabbed in the back by his father and his little brother. As a result, Jack believed the world wasn't a safe place to be in, and he had carried feelings of betrayal with him all his life. Additionally, he had become a fitness junkie in order to bulk up and become invulnerable against his father. As we worked, his pain decreased to the point where he could resume working out and begin to trust others again.

Buried negative emotions relating to chronic or longstanding pain or illness can be disrupting to our energy system. Sometimes we cannot deal with the big feelings or traumatic event at the time it happens, so we bury the experience in our body.

For example, Carrie came to see me for sciatica she'd had for twenty years, and it was now threatening to put her on disability. I asked Carrie when she remembered first feeling a pain like this, and she recalled that it started around the time she left home, when she partnered with a man her mother didn't like. The last thing her mother said to Carrie as she left was, "It's never going to work and you're going to go to hell." What a pain in the butt thing to say.

As we tapped, Carrie became keenly aware of emotions she had never expressed about her mother's words, and that her mom had been a pain in the butt all these years. She tapped on her mom being a literal pain in the butt. As we tapped, her pain was jumping all over the place, in her leg and throughout her body. We kept chasing it. When done, she could walk without pain for the first time in years and was able to continue working full time.

When Sick, Ask Your Immune System to Pay Attention

When you feel sick or at the first hint of a cold or scratchy throat, you might try something I do. It's not Gold Standard EFT per se, but it does involve tapping.

My mentor, Reneé Brown, suggests speaking directly to your immune system and tapping with your requests to feel better. Your body may surprise you in its ability to respond and heal. I ask my immune system to pay special attention to any harmful or unhealthy viruses or infections and the like that are hurting my body right now. I acknowledge the symptoms I am feeling. Then I pair that with a request to the immune system to adjust or reboot, tapping all the way. Here are some of the types of phrases I have used on myself:

> Even though I'm feeling sick, I'm asking my immune system to pay attention to any unwanted infections, invaders, or strange viruses floating through my system and neutralize them.
>
> Even though my throat is all scratchy and sore, I ask my immune system to cool and soothe the mucus membranes in my throat and body.
>
> I'm asking my immune system to step it up a bit, to strengthen and recognize infections that don't belong in my body and increase its function in a gentle, easy, natural, and healing manner, for the entirety of my being and highest good.
>
> Even though my immune system is overreacting to [substance)], I want my body to know that we're safe, and that this is not life-threatening, so we can dial the immune response down a couple notches so I can function.
>
> I'm asking for my body to send soothing, cooling energy to my inflamed joints in a way that is gentle, easy, and kind to my system to release the toxicity. I choose to know that my immune system is healthy, fully functioning, and effectively taking care of this infection. I allow my immune system to balance and quickly zap these viruses, bacteria, parasites, or whatever else does not belong here and is dragging me down for my overall well-being.

Allergies and Tapping

While about 60 percent of my clients are allergic to cats, our cat, Mr. Purr, lives in the home (not in the part that's my office) but none of them have ever had an allergic symptom in the office. I too used to have cat allergy. It's my sense that an allergic reaction in many cases is similar to the overreaction of the phobic (irrational fear) response but the overreaction is diverted to the immune system instead of the nervous system. (See chapter 9 on phobias.) Both have been cleared in my practice with EFT using a similar approach.

I have helped clients resolve smoke, rash, sinus, food, and other allergies with tapping. Practitioners have created entire protocols for allergy clearing with remarkable success rates. I believe that allergies, like phobias, can arise because they are linked with bad experiences the person had while near or involved with the allergen in question. The brilliant primitive brain mistakenly notes anything near the trauma that happened as something to avoid. The phobia affects the nervous system; the allergy affects the immune system.

Tapping on Your Own Symptoms for Sickness or Pain

When you don't know where to start, a great place to begin is asking yourself what was happening in your life just before or during the time you got sick. What was going on with your work, family, social life, spiritual life, relationships, physical body, or any other important area of your life? Major life stressors or big emotional upheavals can be enough to upset the applecart of health.

Sometimes, the emotional origins of the illness are rooted in an incident from a very long time ago that had a serious effect on you but wasn't resolved. For example, Talia wound up very sick after experiencing a significant and traumatic loss. She had a genetically inherited illness she'd had her entire life that had never sidelined her until then. Within about three months of the loss, she went out on disability. We were able to track back significant events and moments during those three months that may have contributed to the issues she was experiencing at the time. We also tapped on three key specific core stories from her childhood. In the next months, she had completely transformed her life—she was at work doing what she loved, volunteering, and once again feeling the many possibilities life had to offer. When you do not even remember the origins of the illness, your body does.

Places to Start Exploring with Chronic and Serious Illnesses

You'll never run out of topics to tap on with this one. These are just a few suggestions.

1. Tap on physical symptoms one at a time with Chase the Pain and see where this takes you. It regularly takes tappers straight to the cause.

2. Ask questions: What was going on, specifically, within a few months before, during, or after the time you got sick? Are there upsetting events or big transitions —losses, moves, job changes, deaths, accidents, divorces, children moving away, vacations that didn't happen, sudden shocks—that you have not worked through yet? Use what you know and tap on any specific events that come up.

If there was an upside to this illness, what might it be? What's the downside of getting better? If there were a reason for this illness no matter how outrageous or crazy it sounds, what might that be (go with first thoughts that come to mind). Take a wild guess and you may uncover a deep-seated unconscious belief from your childhood that you have outgrown. Then you can go to work tapping on that.

When's the first time you felt like this? How does the pain/illness make you feel? Tap on the troublesome feelings relating to experiencing your situation.

3. Explore the belief systems, self-talk, inner critic, fears, and other thoughts you have about being sick or in pain. What do you believe that other people think about you because of the illness?

What stories are you making up in your head about what's going on with you? Are you angry with yourself or others that you're not better? Do you have concerns about not making financial ends meet? Do you believe it's your fault you are sick and that you shouldn't be sick? Are you angry that you don't have the life you planned and envisioned?

4. Tap on upset stemming from hurtful things that happen in your day-to-day life due to your illness, such as hurtful words (or the silent treatment) from well-meaning people who don't get what you're going through. Tap on issues stemming from medical professionals and your care. For example, one client let me know that he taps each time before going to the doctor, while in the waiting room, and after leaving. Tap on specific upsetting events relating to your medical care, problem hospital stays, thoughtless things that hurt, when you looked to a physician or caregiver for hope and instead received nothing encouraging. What sort of prejudice have you experienced? Has your self-worth and status taken a hit?

5. Are you "shoulding" on yourself? It shouldn't be this way. Tap on those shoulds!

6. Are you hating your body because it's causing so much pain? Tap on that. Remember, your body is your partner. Tapping can help you shift your relationship with your body. I can't tell you how many times it's happened in my office that someone who has been at war with their body is overcome with emotion when I suggest we thank his or her body for carrying all this pain for him/her all this time or thank the body for holding up through all of this trouble. It's big and it's deep. It's useful to send some positive messages to your body, too.

7. Tap on the shame, blame, and guilt you have relating to your illness. Do you blame yourself because you should somehow be able to handle everything life throws at you? Do you believe the illness is your fault, somehow?

8. Invoke gratitude. It seems hard to be grateful when you're in pain or feeling miserable, but it seems that's one of the ways out of the pain and misery. The feelings of gratitude and appreciation actually evoke an immune-enhancing response. Even if you don't feel grateful but you feel hateful, pretend. Or look back in your memory for one good experience, something you really appreciated, and savor the memory for at least 12 to 30 seconds. See it, hear it, feel it, really note it—it takes longer for your brain to register the positive. Practice every day. Start a gratitude journal. It takes practice when you are suffering with illness or pain, but you can do it.

Exercise: Tapping in Gratitude for Your Body's Magnificence

Step 1. Start tapping on the points or your favorite point or the finger points now.

Step 2. This exercise offers gratitude for the magnificent body that's carried you around all these years. Try this simple way to begin recognizing how amazing your body is, and shower it with gratitude. Pick one little or big thing you like about your body to start. If you can't think of anything, what about appreciating the fact that your body breathes without you having to do anything?

Step 3. If strong feelings are coming up because you can't find anything to like about your body, this is a great opportunity for you to tap on identifying what you *don't* like and list in your EFT journal any specific incidents that are coming to mind relating to what you don't like about your body.

Tap while taking the time to write down everything that comes to mind about not liking your body. Tap on those aspects one at a time until resistance subsides and just one thing (or more) bubbles up that you do appreciate about your body you are willing to tap on. I understand that when your body is sick, when you have major allergies and have a hard time eating almost any food without a reaction, when your allergy is to something like the sun, or when you have muscle pain no matter what you do, it can be hard to find something to appreciate or that's likable. The body can feel like the enemy even though it's not. You can simply track the pain—or you can tap on tail-enders about finding a positive thing you appreciate about your body. If you thought about something positive and then had a tail-ender, go with that.

Here's some examples: "Even though I don't like my body"; "Even though I find it hard to be grateful when my body doesn't do what I want it to"; "Even though my body isn't doing what it's supposed to do"; "Even though I'm really angry at my body for...."

Remember to rate your intensity before and after tapping the EFT basic recipe. When you are able to think about your body with minimal resistance, you can go to the next step.

Step 4. Tap on the positive body. While I generally don't believe that tapping scripts will get at the roots of an individual's unique issue, they are often a good starting point to find hidden treasure, paving the way to finding out what's underneath a certain negative behavior or thought pattern. Here's a tapping script by one of my favorite tappers, Brad Yates, who offers hundreds of YouTube tapping videos on just about every subject possible, including insomnia—in which he greets viewers with sleep cap. [23]

Brad has kindly allowed me to share his tapping script below. What follows is just one part. As you know, scripts may not get you to the deep center of your own issues relating to pain and illness, but they may inspire in other ways.

> ***Karate chop:*** I choose to feel really good. I really love and accept myself. Love and forgive myself. Choose to feel physically great. Vibrant health and well-being are my birthright.

---

23. Brad Yates, "Tapping Into Vibrant Health," YouTube, accessed January 11, 2015, www.youtube.com/watch?v=Ar1G_cnL_T4 (Script: www.vidqt.com/id/Ar1G_cnL_T4?lang=en&kind=asr).

And there's some stuff getting in the way, and I choose to let that go. I choose to feel really good, and I deeply and completely love, and forgive and accept myself.

Tapping on the points starting with the top of the head and moving down through all the points—one phrase, one point: I am grateful, body, for all the ways you keep me going. (Maybe less is more here): You keep me going, you breathe without my even reminding you, digest all my food and send it around to where it's needed, tell me when I need to rest.

Truly, my body is a work of art, a miracle, and I am grateful to have life in a body, and everything that means to me. I love my body— or I'd like to! I am grateful to my body for all the ways and all the times it has carried and supported me. Thank you, thank you, thank you.

Repeat this exercise anytime you need a boost.

In Conclusion

Now you have some great tools to begin tapping on the physical, whether you're recovering from an acute injury, the common cold, from an accident, or navigating life with a serious illness. In the next chapter we address how to put phobias in their place, which is no place in your body or mind.

Chapter 9
Neutralizing Phobias

After being assaulted by a would-be purse-snatcher in the parking lot of a local grocery store, Eliana was dragged nearly 75 feet. Her injuries were painful, but as Eliana said, "Far worse was the fear that overtook me. At first I wasn't even aware of it, but a few days after the event, I realized I was in trouble."

Eliana began to imagine being attacked everywhere she went. She tried talk therapy for several months but it didn't seem to help. "I could hardly step outside the door to feed the cat because I feared another attack."

About nine months after the attack, she learned about EFT. "I started tapping and within ten minutes, the fear was gone! The contrast between the long hours of talk therapy that did little for me and the swift resolution from EFT was astonishing. I then used EFT on the residual pain from my injuries. EFT was more effective than the prescription painkiller my doctor had ordered."

Eliana's fast phobic resolution is not uncommon. As is the case with her example, some phobic responses can be traced to one event. The phobias resolve quite quickly as a result and are called "one-minute wonders" in the EFT world.

When your reaction to a stimulus is disproportionate to the actual danger posed and you'll go to extreme lengths to avoid your fear target, that's a phobia. Using EFT to eliminate phobic responses or panic has been quite effective in my own personal and professional lives. In my professional practice, young children have released phobias that include fear of tornados, school, speaking up in class, and even fear of bowel movements after diarrhea. Adults have cleared phobias that include fear of public speaking, social anxiety, elevators, dentists, doctors, heights, water, driving, airplane travel, stairs and escalators, insects and snakes, and claustrophobia.

Tapping doesn't remove your notions of safety and common sense. It resolves the energy disruption at the heart of your mind-body's excessive response to the specific stimulus causing you to involuntarily overreact. More than 11 percent of people will have a phobia at some point in their lives.[24] The percentage is likely higher, as those with phobias often keep their problem a secret, reporting privately that they are ashamed.

How Do Phobias Start?

At the heart of your fear response is a disruption in your body's energy system. Recall the Discovery Statement from chapter 1: "The cause of all negative emotions is a disruption in the body's energy system." In the case of phobia, something you experienced hurt or scared you. You experienced an energy disruption, according to EFT. Your "primitive" brain took control to keep you safe from danger. Your phobic reaction alert is ongoing in your remarkable limbic brain, whose amazing memory cache is much like RAM on your computer. That is, the mind will keep reacting to the original threat in the same way until you are able to resolve the energy disruption from the initial trauma. This is why each time you come in

24. Heather Hatfield, "The Fear Factor: Phobia," WebMD, accessed January 15, 2015, www.webmd.com/anxiety-panic/guide/fear-factor-phobias.

contact with or anywhere near the fearful target, your protector and survival-focused brain is saying, "Danger! Danger! Stay away!" That's why you haven't been able to do anything—until today.

It might be useful for you to tap while you read. You can try tapping continuously on the fingertip points, starting with the tip of the thumb, index finger, third finger, and pinkie. Or tap the gamut point, between the ring and pinkie on the top of the hand just behind the knuckles. Why not move that life force right on through?

People with phobias can't imagine coming into contact with their fear-object, let alone resolving the phobia itself. With EFT, you are in control of just how far you'll go toward resolving your phobia. You stop as soon as you experience a bit of discomfort and tap.

You know by now that when you get specific about the events and the aspects underneath them, you will access the actual emotional and experiential contributors sustaining the phobic response. Apply the EFT basic recipe one round at a time to each individual aspect of your fear.

What if you don't remember how and when the big fear started? Your subconscious will do the work, accessing the deeper specific feelings and issues under the phobia. If you need to know how the phobia started, the event *will* come to mind, with patience. If you don't need to know, you won't know how it started, but you will still neutralize your phobia. You can use the stimulus itself as your target. Either way, it works.

Case Study: Fear of Flying Neutralized

Ali had a fear of flying for as long as she could remember. She said, "In college, when my parents offered to send airfare for me to fly the five hundred miles home on a 45-minute plane trip, I chose the 8-hour bus ride. I didn't want to get on a small plane. I didn't want to die that way. That's how scared I was."

As she regularly had to travel overseas for her work and to visit friends and family, flying was as much of a trauma for her flight-mates as it was for her! As Ali explained it, she was a terrible person to sit next to. She wouldn't get up during the flight. She white-knuckled from clenching so tight, had visions of crashing the entire time the plane was in the air, and turbulence compelled her to grab the person next to her, stranger or not.

Things came to a head when Ali received notice from her work that in five weeks her job would require her to fly to four different destinations in a two-week time span. Having recently learned EFT she thought: "This is going to be okay. I'm going to tap on this."

At the time she was involved in an online tapping group, so she announced to the group her intentions, gathering support. She had five weeks to resolve this lifelong phobia. She started like so: "Even though just thinking about this upcoming flight I feel panic, I deeply and completely accept myself."

Then she tapped several times daily whenever she thought of the upcoming trips, on every single specific aspect that came up: "Even though I can't breathe, there's not enough air; I don't know if the pilot will have been drinking; I hate air travel; I don't like that I can't tell what's going on; I have no control"and so on. She tapped until she felt no intensity thinking about any part of the travel, from arriving at the airport to landing.

The true test came on flight day. "I remember looking at the plane, stepping onto the plane, and realizing my 'radar' was not going out of control." Her next thought was that she was hungry and she wondered what they would serve on the flight. Food hadn't been part of the picture in the past. Once in the air, she reports, "Instead of all the negative racing thoughts, I was curious about what was going on around me. Looking out the window, I remembering thinking, 'this is romantic, this is wonderful.'" At that point, she could still remember how the panic felt, but she didn't have it. "I used to book a flight and start praying. Now I just think I used to be afraid to fly. I don't have that anymore!"

In that above case, Ali didn't know the origins of the phobia, and it didn't matter. In the case that follows, there was an originating event.

Case Study: Debbie and Fear of Stairs

Often one thing becomes linked with another, eliciting a phobic response. Debbie, age 45, was terrified of walking down but not up stairs. She had no memory of a time when it didn't feel like she was going to die when she had to walk downstairs; she had inched her way down stairs in terror her whole life. We started at the top of five stories of stairs and tapped on all aspects—every possible thought, feeling, sensation, and belief—keeping her from walking down one single stair. Aspects included: can't look down, nothing there, need to hold on, and more. After about ten minutes she took a single step on her own. But then she wouldn't release her grip on the railing. "I'll fall," she said. We had uncovered another aspect. We tapped now on aspects relating to releasing her death grip on the railing. Then, we stepped back to the top. Now, I asked her to look down, imagine walking with the hand off the railing, to get her tuned back into the falling fear. I then asked her what the falling fear reminded her of.

As is common in situations with EFT, an early memory surfaced from when she was five years old. Her family was hiking down a craggy bluff, with Debbie lagging behind. Her parents were in front of her and arguing loudly. Debbie had felt alone, scared, and uncomfortable, and she was also quite close to the edge of the rocky hill. Shortly after that event, her parents divorced. Being high up on the hill looking down while her parents argued had been very scary, and it was the last time the family went on an outing together. Somehow, the fear of going down the hill had generalized to going down regular stairs, crowded stairs, stairs with no railing and the like, and they had been tightly linked ever since. But really, she had just been scared about her parents arguing so heatedly and linked it to the big loss of her father's regular presence and love. Once we resolved this issue, I had a feeling she would be able to walk down stairs, and I was right. But were we done?

Soon after we felt "complete," a whole group of people entered the stairwell and her fear spiked. Now we tapped on the aspect of crowded stairwells. She was walking up and down stairs "just like a regular person," no fear. The next session we went to steep, metal fire escape stairs to scan for aspects and test our results. In fact, I was the one who had to tap on my fear of the metal stairs! Ali was practically giddy with excitement she was so happy to feel free of the fear that had haunted her all these years. She had unlinked decades of terror and fear in just two sessions.

Exercise: Overcoming Phobia: Get Curious, Ask Questions

When you clear a phobia target with tapping, your questions will be like guideposts to direct your tapping. Note that the following questions may look familiar to you, as they are the same types of questions we apply to just about any bothersome problem. List them and your answers in your EFT journal. They will help you uncover aspects and specific events to tap on.

- When and where did my phobic response start? Who was with me?
- What was going on in my life at the time?
- When did the fear get worse?
- Do I remember a time that I didn't have it?
- What does this fear feeling remind me of?
- When do/did I remember having a feeling similar to this?
- How ashamed am I of the phobia?
- Am I keeping my phobia a secret? What will happen if I tell someone?
- What happens when I tell other people about my phobia?

- What do I believe about myself because of the phobia?
- Do I have a case of the "shoulds"? You know the self-talk/inner critic: "I should not have," "I'm wrong to have," "I'm bad to have this," "I'm a loser to have this," etc.
- What happens when I see, hear, feel, touch, taste, or think of my fear target?
- What are my body sensations when I think or come near my fear target? Does your breathing get shallow and fast? Is your chest tight, does your gut feel like it's going to clench into a fist, are your legs trembling, can you not seem to get enough air?

How Long Will It Take?

You might be wondering how long it will take you to clear your phobia. Everyone is different. You may clear the root of your phobia in five minutes of tapping and resolve the problem for good. Or it may take many rounds—or even many days—to have a breakthrough. There may be hundreds of aspects and several specific events you'll need to tap on before your phobia clears. Be persistent. You can heal this. You will likely need to put yourself in the fear situation at some point to truly test for results. Working with a practitioner can be especially useful in situations like these.

Suggestions for Working through Phobias

Look at your phobia as if it were an archeological site; do a little digging, and you will see many civilizations buried one on top of another. Remove them one at a time and you will unearth everything you need to know to clear your fear. If you have a fear of saying a target word, such as "snake," tap on "the s-word," for example. Or you can use a code word that has nothing to do with the phobia itself, like "my bunny friend," or "the Tesla factor," or "the big yuck." If you feel ready, you can start to tap on saying the name of your fear target out loud and tapping on the intensity that just saying it elicits. Do this until you can actually say out loud the name of your fear target with neutrality or something close to it. If you can't get there, then you may find working with a practitioner experienced in helping clients resolve phobias useful.

Exercise: Taking the Edge Off Just Thinking of the Target

Step 1. *I cannot even think of my fear target without upset.* If this speaks to you, start there, at this outermost layer. Tap until you no longer feel triggered and resistant when just thinking about the fear target. This is similar to the Tearless Trauma technique, approaching the most global perspective possible to take the edge off and be as comfortable as possible.

Try customizing any one of these phrases to suit your own situation:

> Even though I feel trapped, I deeply and completely love and accept myself.
>
> Even though this fear has control over me, I deeply and profoundly love and accept myself anyway.
>
> Even though there's a lot here, and I don't know where to start, I deeply and completely accept myself.
>
> Even though I'm terrified of certain things, I accept my terror and myself.
>
> Even if I never get over this, I still love and accept myself anyway (or that's okay).

Step 2. Remember to rate your intensity on just thinking about this issue before creating your setup phrase, then karate chop: "Even though I don't even want to think about the fear I have, I deeply and profoundly accept myself anyway." Now tap down the points with your reminder phrase "don't even want to think about it," and retest your intensity again, just about that one aspect of thinking about it.

Step 3. Once you have tapped that down to a neutral intensity and have no resistance to thinking about the fear object, continue by tapping on every single aspect that comes to mind, using the ratings scale as your feedback loop. The most important factor is to not get ahead of yourself but take things one step at a time. If you push or rush past a detail that has not been tapped down to zero, you are hampering your own efforts to resolve the issue.

Exercise: Fill in the Blanks

Here are a few more options for tapping around the edges of a phobia. These are the types of statements I have used in my own practice, but you can certainly create your own. These are a phobia's related thoughts and beliefs:

Even though I'll never get over this fear of ______________ (e.g., escalators), I am still a good person.

Even though I'm ______________(e.g., scared), I deeply and completely accept myself.

Even though I am ______________(e.g., tired of living in fear of this phobia)....

Even though I've had this for______________(e.g., ten years), I'm open to the possibility of healing this fear today.

Even though I want to get over this ______________(e.g., water phobia) but don't yet know how, I deeply and profoundly accept myself and I'm open to healing it.

If you find you're unable or unwilling to take the next steps, it may mean coming into contact with the fear target still provokes too much fear for you to easily handle. For those who have suffered significant trauma in their lives, it is not recommended you do this on your own. Do not go a step further than you feel absolutely comfortable with. Don't give yourself grief; get relief.

Reframes: Choosing Differently Around Your Fear after Clearing Intensity

You can ask yourself to make different choices, once you have cleared a significant amount of intensity relating to the phobic response. You'll know you're ready for some reframes if they make sense now, or if other options start to come to mind of their own accord. You might consider asking yourself, "How would I rather experience this X that I used to be afraid of?" Or, "What would feel better than the way that I used to be around this X?"

When new choices or reframes work, you can completely saturate yourself in the new way of thinking or considering.

Even though…I choose to experience this differently from now on.

Even though…I'd rather experience peace even if I never get over this.

Even though…what if I could see this differently?

Even though…I wonder how it would feel to be calm?

Even though…I choose to see that this is really no threat to me.

Even though…what if it won't really kill me? That's a novel thought!

Even though…I see that my life isn't in danger after all!

Even though…it's such a relief to experience neutrality around X.

Even though…I choose to be calm and confident.

Testing Your Results

After you've tapped down your intensity to zero, you will want to put yourself into the fear situation if possible to test your results. And if another aspect arises, use it! As happened with Debbie and shedding the stair fear, another aspect may arise when you are faced with a new trigger that you haven't covered in your tapping. For instance, perhaps an elevator with glass doors will spike intensity, when all other elevators have no charge. Or maybe spiders that are larger than your fist will spike intensity, while all others don't bother you at all. Just tap on the intensity of this new aspect until it, too, collapses. Yes, your unreasonable (and whatever else you call them in your mind) limiting fears can be conquered!

Case Study: Public Speaking Phobia

I have worked with many people to neutralize one of the most common phobias, public speaking. In each case, the phobia was held up by early childhood events, such as a move to a new home and school when the child was not ready, needing to be loyal to an introverted sibling, being singled out at a very young age for too much public attention, and so on.

Fifteen-year-old Maggie was attending boarding school far away from her family. Just three years earlier, Maggie had been an outgoing, well-liked girl at the top of her seventh grade class. She had "contracted" some social phobias about the time of her family's move to a new home. The slight shyness had by age fifteen turned into social and public speaking phobias that were running her life. She couldn't even speak to two people without fear, anxiety, and panic. Speaking up and answering questions in class was troublesome for her. The worst was that she had to do a public debate for one of her classes, once a month.

During winter break, while Maggie visited the family, her mother signed her on to tap with me. For her part, Maggie was not thrilled, but she was cautiously willing to try anything to get over the fear she had. We started with general tapping as I gathered information. The worst part for her was the school's monthly public speaking debate. We tackled every single aspect of this: what happened when she went to the debate, her self-talk, and the feelings she had. She tapped on: *feeling stupid, dumb, helpless; losing my voice; feeling like I'm going to faint; humiliation and shame; can't speak, can't breathe; standing there with the paper unable to see the words; the subjects to debate are boring; I hate that class*—until they were all neutralized.

The true test would come only when she returned to school some two weeks later.

The day after our session, Maggie went to a party. She reported with surprise that where she normally would have hidden in a corner, she was comfortable opening up, speaking to friends, and meeting new people. Her experience motivated her to continue.

In our next session, we tapped on every aspect that happened for her leading up to a debate. We started with her being in the classroom just before the debate. We tapped again on all her feelings and self-talk: *dread; knowing it was going to happen again; feeling helpless; wanting to be anywhere but there; knowing I was going to look stupid and mess up; feeling hopeless; the long walk down the hall to the classroom; the other kids I had to debate; I didn't like the speech; I didn't feel ready; I won't be able to open my mouth; I might faint.* When she could think of no more upsets around the upcoming event, we moved on to what happens after the debate, tapping on all the thoughts, feelings, and body sensations we could drum up, even though she was not yet in the real situation.

A couple of times I asked her about when the whole issue had gotten worse; everything pointed to the move and the change in schools. She explained to me that one moment in particular stood out. It was in French class, where she was asked to speak up, and she couldn't understand what she was being asked and was humiliated. In her old school, she had been ahead; but here she felt hopelessly behind. We naturally applied Tell the Story to this event: "The Awful French." Finally, the upset around the event cleared. The sound of her voice had shifted as we tapped from soft, to loud, to slow, to angry—a common occurrence with tapping, I had an intuition that the phobia was more than just French class; the word "anger" kept coming to me. For me, these intuitions are like little prompts or arrows saying "Try this! Say that!" Maybe intuition is just the combined sum of experience, the ability to see, listen, integrate, and synthesize information quickly. In any case, I use caution when saying these things, so I pre-frame my thoughts to the client (this is a common EFT practice, by the way): "This may not have anything to do with your situation, or it may be spot-on, but I'm going to say it to you and you tell me if this lands or makes any sense."

Listen to your own intuition as well as your logic. The way things are sometimes linked in the subconscious sometimes makes no logical sense, but following the trail leads to relief. Maggie came in touch with the fact that she was really angry at her mother because of all the things she had missed out on due to the family moving such as: not graduating at the top of her seventh grade class with all her friends, grieving that she didn't get to stay good-bye, and not having any choice in the matter of switching schools. Her natural anger with her mother over the enforced move was the piece that finally caused the whole public speaking issue to cave. The mother reported that the next day Maggie had expressed a surprising amount of anger at her. We tapped on the mother's guilt for "making" the family move. When Maggie later returned to school, she debated. The panic, phobia, and social anxiety were gone! Some two years later, Maggie's still happily phobia-free.

EFT for Allergies

We discussed allergies in chapter 8, but it's worth bringing up here again. It's my sense that an allergic reaction in many cases is similar to the overreaction of the phobic response, but the over-reaction is diverted to the immune system instead of to the nervous system.

In Conclusion

Fear builds on itself. That's the brilliance of our survival-tuned mind. You can change things, and when you do, the fear dissolves as if it had never been. Now you know how to resolve phobias and panic by tapping on feelings and bodily symptoms as well as the root of the fear.

In the next chapter, we take a look at weight and body issues and self-esteem.

Chapter 10
Weight Release, Cravings, and Body Confidence

My tapping buddy Zoe had cravings she felt were beyond her control: the specific café she could not pass without stopping for a mocha, sugary snacks, especially chocolates; candy on sale; and diet cola. Like most people with cravings or addictions, she was high-functioning and kept this shadow side on the down-low. She was ashamed of her lack of control and of herself. Self-shame is a great way to lock in an unhelpful behavior.

Zoe was an entrepreneur, doing very well for herself. She had a healing practice on the side, and led an active social, church, and volunteer life. She was health conscious, loving, generous, optimistic, and upbeat... but had been enslaved by these cravings for decades. So what was up with all the cravings? Zoe felt ready to look at what was underneath the cravings, deal with it, and let the whole thing go!

Cravings like Zoe's are not uncommon. Many of us have areas of our lives where we cannot control our behavior around a substance, a person, or a situation. Some of us pretend we're in control when we're really not. Yet we are getting our needs met in the best ways we know how. Many of these behavioral craving patterns go back to events from childhood. What is underneath the behavior? Could it be an unmet, deep-seated need, such as the need for love, the need for comfort, the need for safety? A feeling and situation that is very painful to us that we don't believe we have the resources to deal with? In any case, there are times when we don't even know we're hurting.

It took me years to connect the dots and understand that my urge to stop at garage sales after doing deep emotional work meant that I was hurting and displacing emotions that were still processing. It was the best solution I had at the time for big hurts, but man did I get some awesome stuff! Coping isn't all bad, is it?

What are your solutions? I'm not referring to turning to healthy sources for support and help when you feel off-track. I'm talking about solutions that may look like excessive alcohol or drug addiction. Sometimes it's hookup sex or Internet porn; sometimes it's sweet things or carbs; sometimes it's a certain type of relationship drama; sometimes it's work-a-holism. We numb because we are about to feel our "difficult" emotions, which we haven't been taught to feel and thus aren't willing. We are disconnecting even though we are lonely and need connection. This loop is not useful as a long-term solution.

In this chapter, we're picking at the tip of the iceberg on some compelling topics—clearing food cravings, taking a look at what's underneath weight-release issues, and experiencing body confidence. You'll come away with some suggestions and exercises to gain self-confidence about your glorious body. Did that phrase "your glorious body" activate some intensity for you? Tap. Notice where you feel resistance in your body, too. You can also tap a round on that. You can just tap on your fingertips, or select one point and gently massage it, or Tarzan tap. Or you can run an EFT round like this, checking intensity before and after tapping:

> Even though I feel upset just thinking about all my trouble with (cravings/with my body) and (how I look/body part),

I deeply and completely love, honor, accept, and forgive myself and anyone else who contributed to this upset in any way.

As you already know, the takeaway here is that you can tap on whatever you're feeling. Know that the feelings, emotions, and body sensations are tied to a past event, remembered or long-forgotten. And even if you don't know the events, you have the feelings that will help you clear the energy disruption and the today issue—the craving or body hatred.

Let yourself feel the feelings and watch them wash through you so they can go on their merry way. It may be challenging, especially if you have a backlog of unresolved painful upsets. I remind myself regularly when things start to spin out of control: "you are having feelings; they are not doing anything *to* you, you're simply *experiencing* them." You are not a victim of your feelings. They are simply information, and they help. If the feelings don't subside or you consistently feel like you are drowning in them but can't find your way back to shore, consider working with a trustworthy practitioner or mental health professional.

How about tapping on or massaging the collarbone point right now, or tap the finger points and then the gamut points as you read?

Underneath the Carbs, the Coffee, the Cravings

We eat when we're happy. We eat when we're sad. We eat out of habit. We eat to fill a need somehow not being met. When we have cravings, we're just trying to take care of ourselves in the best way we know. What if we're stuck in a cycle of coping behavior that perhaps worked well once but is not working so well anymore? What if we have the resources and tools to handle whatever is underneath our craving—more resources than we did when we took on the coping pattern as a solution to a problem? We only need to reboot the part of our body-mind system that is freaking out for the craving—and feel the feelings underneath. You track an addiction back; underneath the compulsion, feelings, and sensations is a memory (sometimes a good one, sometimes a bad one) associated with the object of the craving or addiction.

Aim Gold Standard EFT at enough core events and their associated aspects underlying the craving, and the entire issue resolves. The emotion is disconnected from the crave object or unhealthy behavior—the whole thing dissolves.

Case Study: Zoe's Cravings

With Zoe, we started addressing her cravings for Cocoa Kisses from Hershey's, and later we also took care of her Russell Stover fixation. With this work, her entire issue collapsed. It generalized to other candy and sweets cravings—remember the Generalization Effect—so she no longer had the sweet cravings and ice cream marathon challenges.

We started the work slowly. I had her put the chocolates she craved in the other room, where she couldn't even see them. Just thinking about them, Zoe wanted one of those candies at a level of 10. We tapped on her feeling of wanting it, including where in her body she was feeling this "wanting," which turned out to be in her chest. We tapped on both the body sensation and the wanting until the feeling and sensation subsided.

Then I asked her to get a piece of chocolate from the other room and only look at it. Now she wanted it again, at a 10—or in her words, "a bazillion." One specific aspect was its appearance. Zoe remarked on its "pretty blue metallic wrapping paper; it's like a little present!"

For my part, my brain got very perky, busy making associations. I remembered Zoe had received a lot of presents from her father, who had died years earlier. Could the "Cocoa Kiss Compulsion" have something to do with that? We tapped on the beautiful present aspect until her "bazillion" was neutralized to zero. We tapped on the feeling of tightness in her body when she thought she couldn't have it but wanted it so much. This, too, subsided to zero.

However, now the big feelings about missing her father and the way he had doted on her skyrocketed in intensity in both her body sensations and feelings about him. We tapped several rounds on different aspects of her missing him until she was able to talk about it with neutrality. Paying attention to intuition is important with EFT.

I asked Zoe to simply hold the candy in her hand without unwrapping it. Again, we tapped on the increase in the "wanting" intensity. When that subsided, I asked her to unwrap the little kiss. She hesitated—she didn't want to open it and not eat it, it would be wasted. We tapped on her concern about wasting things, which had been another theme in her growing-up years. We then tapped on the smell of the chocolate, on the fact that they were on sale, and like her father before her, she had *always* bought candy on sale. She had associated candy on sale with receiving gifts from her father and the great love she experienced as a result.

We tapped on the fact that she gave much of this candy away to the kids in her dance studio and to strangers on the street. We tapped on how good it felt to give these presents away to others, how "sweet" it was. We tapped on her need to please others and then how she couldn't just eat one but had to eat a whole bag. We tapped on how bad all this sugar actually was for her. We tapped on every sensual aspect of the candy that gave her intensity.

Then we tapped on her own self-talk/inner critic related to the candy: "I am a pig. I am a glutton. I am not honoring my body. This is disgusting. I am ashamed. What's wrong with me?"

You might think that because I was a friend of hers, I would have said something to quickly reassure her: "No, you're not disgusting and you're not a pig! I really admire you." But that's exactly what she *didn't* need—one more person to *not* listen to her. I needed to validate her feelings and listen to her without being judgmental to support her as she moved through her craving addiction. She needed to work through all the negative aspects first. I knew she wasn't those things she was calling herself, but I needed to meet her at the point where she was standing, not where *I* wanted her to be.

Throughout this round of tapping, I continually checked and rechecked how she was feeling about wanting the candy in the moment. Zoe's need was subsiding as we tapped down all the aspects relating to the craving.

Sometime during this process, it came to mind that her father had especially given her approval when she was giving love away to others (which later led us to another core issue that was resolved). She came to understand that by purchasing the candy, she was trying to recreate that loving, safe relationship she had as a child with her father. "I wanted to be loved in that same way, and the candy was helping me recreate the feeling."

Her craving disappeared, never to return. We asked her brain networking to rewire so that she no longer needed to access the loving memories of her father through these candies—she could have the love and good memories with her all the time. This is a variation of Gold Standard EFT. (As you know, even Gold Standard founder Gary Craig is, as of this writing, exploring a form of EFT—Optimal EFT—that doesn't involve tapping at all.) Zoe and I tapped for letting candy be candy and love be an emotion, two separate and distinct things, not mixed together anymore.

Here are a few paraphrases of our setups for tapping rounds:

> Even though I love this candy, I am choosing to let candy be candy and love be love. Even though I have associated candy with love, I now know candy is just a piece of colored sugar and has nothing to do with the love I feel for my father and the love he shared with me.

Even though Dad isn't with me now, I can feel this good feeling anytime I think of him; I no longer need candy to experience this deep love.

I'm asking my brain circuitry to redo and reboot so all parts of me know and live from the space that love and candy are no longer connnected. I no longer need candy to experience the love. I can experience that at anytime.

After about forty-five minutes, she had no desire for the candy. In fact, when she did taste it (I requested that she taste it—you always need to test or how will you really know?), she didn't want it. It no longer even tasted good to her! She never looked back, either, and the craving never resurfaced.

Exercise: Getting Curious about Cravings

We're going to focus on cravings for food (the ones you can't control), although the directions can apply to any type of addiction. Use the craved object as your target when you review the questions in the exercise below.

Step 1. Start tapping now as you work. Why harbor unnecessary upset? As you read, tap down the points, from the top of the head through the under arm point. You can also tap on your fingertips or hold the palm of your hand against a particular point and massage that area as you read.

Step 2. In your EFT journal create a heading: "Cravings." List any cravings that come to mind. Choose just one to start.

If just writing your list you feel yourself getting upset or falling into a crave hole, stop right there. As Buddhist teacher Tara Brach says, "soften" around the upset, rather than shun it. And start tapping, of course. Use the Tarzan tap, the fingertip taps, or any other point you like. You can also tap a Gold Standard EFT basic recipe on the feelings that have been stimulated, allowing the intensity to subside before moving on. As I have indicated before, use your judgment about accessing additional support as you navigate the exercises.

What if you were curious about your craving, instead of angry, ashamed, or some other challenging emotion?

- What benefits are you receiving from the craving? For example: It's my pacifier. It makes me feel better. I love it. It helps me feel connected. It soothes me. I get distracted so I don't have to think about all my problems.
- What don't you want to see, feel, experience, or think about that results in the craving? Is it to soothe, cover up, or distract yourself from another issue? For example: It tastes good. It takes my attention away from my loneliness. It distracts me from how much I hate my job. It helps me forget how miserable my life is. I don't have to think about....
- Are there specific times of day when cravings rise? After work, once the kids are in bed, after a stressful encounter? What about at bedtime when the house is quiet? Perhaps it's at the gym when you see skinny people and compare yourself unfavorably. Or are there physical triggers, like the smell of fresh pastries at your favorite store, or the aroma of coffee? Consider visual triggers too: driving by the candy store, the pastry shop, even the gas station.
- Are there certain situations, past events, or people who seem to trigger your craving?
- What memories are associated with the craving? They can be positive or negative. For example, someone with a carb and bread craving remembers that her grandmother used to bake fresh bread. She remembers her grandma's kindness and the safety she felt, and she associates both with the smell of the bread. She craves that feeling, that comfort. Someone else might associate a bad memory with their crave object.

He may remember the time his father used to knock him around calling him a dummy; the food displaced the emotional pain.

- When's the first time you felt this craving feeling? What was happening in your life or the life of your family when you first experienced the craving? What does this crave feeling remind you of?

Allow yourself to imagine how would your life be different if you were craving-free and had power over the craving. Write down how your life would be different. Imagine a day in your new life if you can. And remember, no one is making you give it up until you are good and ready. If this part is too painful, let it be for now and return to it once you have tapped on more crave aspects.

The answers to the previous questions are fodder for your tapping. What are the drivers of your cravings? If they are helping you hold up a part of your life that you are otherwise extremely unhappy with, you may need to experience some uncomfortable feelings. Tapping will help you uncover this.

The idea is that once the feelings underneath that craving are neutralized, the disturbance in the body's energy system will also be resolved. The cravings then disappear. In fact, many clients often say the same thing: "I don't even like that food/drink/snack now! It doesn't even taste good." Be prepared. I didn't think I had an unhealthy attitude toward dark chocolate, but after tapping with clients on clearing their cravings, I lost my desire for it!

Step 3. Please note that if you are feeling overwhelmed, like you are doing something wrong and that it's impossible for you to ever get over this, or you've tapped on these feelings but are still feeling negative thoughts and feelings, or complete dissociation, all this means is that you have brought up big stuff. You likely need help navigating through it. Congratulate yourself instead of beating yourself up, and then take the next step of getting the support of an EFT expert or a mental health professional to help you through it. All you need are compassion and care as you touch on old, deep hurts.

Exercise: Clearing Specific Food Cravings

As you read instructions, please start tapping on one of your favorite tapping points. Do this continuously until it's time for a whole round of EFT basic recipe. You can also use the exercises and questions in this chapter to apply to other addictive substances, obsessions, behaviors, and the like. And you can return to these exercises again and again, getting something new each time from them.

Step 1. Get your EFT journal, and choose one food or treat you turn to for cravings. Is it in the house? Ideally, you would have the crave-object in the house. Actually, this type of tapping works best when the object of desire is right in front of you. Be specific! If it's Lay's Original potato chips or Ben and Jerry's Chubby Hubby ice cream or big bags of gluten-free raw dried kale whatever, obtain whatever you crave the most, not the discount knock-off brand. This way you'll get more bang for your buck. And if you are resistant to clearing the craving or somehow afraid about what's going to happen, or that you won't be able to handle it, or that you don't really want to do this, or you don't believe this will work, or there's just so much that's wrong with you, or you're afraid to let this go for fear of what's underneath it, then tap on all of that before moving on to step 2 with the crave object itself. This is called clearing resistance, like getting the snow off the ice rink so you can skate smoothly. Remember, we're all human; there's a lot to heal. And it sure feels good when you're choosing to connect with yourself. Just for the heck of it, can you remember a time when you felt closely connected to yourself and the world? Did it involve a crave object? Probably not.

Step 2. You can start with the crave object in another room, across the room, or on a table in front of you, or even resting in your lap or hand. If just thinking about the crave object brings you up to a 10 on the intensity scale, start there. Let's say the crave object is right in front of you. Rate how much you want your crave object, on the 0 to 10 scale. Write down your number. Where in your body do you feel that wanting, and how intense is the feeling? Write that number down too. While you don't need to tap specifically on your body feeling relating to the craving, you do want to check in regularly about where it has moved and if it has subsided or increased in intensity as you tap on the crave object.

Step 3. Now that you have an intensity number, you can give the crave object a nickname or a title if you so desire, such as "The Seducer," or "My Ruin," or "The Sweet." Go ahead and perform the EFT basic recipe focused on the general wanting of the crave object. Apply tapping until your desire goes down to a manageable level where you are not feeling impelled. If you need to tap through several rounds to get there, do so.

We'll use the example of M&Ms as the crave object. Please customize this EFT setup to reflect your own specific craving. Remember, the EFT basic recipe includes the setup statement as well as the tapping down of the points or the EFT sequence from the top of the head down through under the arm.

Repeat while tapping on the Karate Chop point one to three times: "Even though I want these M&Ms now, I deeply and completely accept myself." Try the reminder phrase "want these M&Ms now." Additionally, if you have located a specific place or guessed at where in your body you are feeling this wanting, you can create a tapping round and run through the basic recipe like so: "Even though I feel this big wanting in my chest (or wherever you feel it—in the throat or like nausea in the stomach), I deeply and completely accept myself."

These examples of EFT setup phrases will give you ideas about where a person can go. Please note that each would be one round of EFT—it's a setup statement, tapping down the points, and testing (and retesting) intensity. Here are more setups for your inspiration:

> Even though a part of me must have these M&Ms right now, I deeply and completely love and accept myself. (Forgive, myself, love myself, honor myself…)
>
> Even though a part of me needs them right this second, that's okay. I choose peace.
>
> Even though I can't bear the thought of this one little treat being taken away from me because I have so little I enjoy in my life….

Consider exaggerating—or it may feel to you like this is no exaggeration:

> Even though it feels like I won't survive without these M&Ms in my life….
>
> Even though a part of me thinks I'll die if I don't get these M&Ms right now….
>
> Even though I'm drawn to them the way a vampire is drawn to blood….

Or power struggle with the rebel inside:

> Even though I'm never going to give them up, and you can't make me, I love myself just as I am….
>
> Even though I'll die if I have to give them up, please don't make me give them up….

Step 4. After performing a round with one or more EFT sequences from the top of the head to under the arm with the reminder or problem phrase, test how much you want your crave object (the M&Ms) and if the body sensation relating to it has changed. If the craving has subsided to below a 2, it's time to take the next step. Otherwise, keep tapping on the general, overall craving until it dips below a 2 before moving on.

Step 4a. Sometimes, the craving won't drop because too many aspects are flooding your mind all at once. Then ask yourself what is one thing that jumps out about how much you want the M&Ms and tap on that one thing only. Stay completely focused on just that one aspect until it subsides. If you do not experience a decrease in your intensity, ask yourself what is in the way. What's the upside of keeping the craving? Tap on that. You may also consider just setting it aside until later and starting again, or you could come at it from a different angle. And of course, you always have the option to obtain the support of an EFT practitioner experienced in clearing cravings.

Step 5. If you have dropped down below a 2 after tapping on the first round, ask yourself about the next quality that jumps out at you about your crave object that makes you want it? It could be a positive or a negative. Here's what comes to mind when looking at the M&Ms bag: "the bag is ugly but the colors inside are so bright and shiny." Notice that these are technically three different aspects (ugly bag, bright colors, shiny colors). When you have several aspects like this that are so closely linked, you could combine them or start with one of these aspects—the highest one—then go for the other two once that one subsides. Probably one round would do it on each. Now rate your intensity of feeling about each quality on the 0 to 10 scale.

Step 6. Let's say you want to combine "bright" and "shiny colors." Create a setup phrase focusing on these qualities. For the M&Ms, it would be: "Even though the colors inside are so bright and shiny and I want them, I deeply and completely accept myself." You would then repeat your EFT setup one to three times while continuously tapping on your Karate Chop point. Again, identify where in your body you feel this, you might say: Even though the colors inside are so bright and shiny and I feel this in my trembling arms . . . .

Step 7. Go to work on the tap-down points, from the top of the head to the underarm point using your reminder or problem phrase. (In the case of the M&Ms: "Bright and shiny colors—I want them!") This might also be a time to try tapping on the finger points and the Nine Gamut series. You'll find these additional tapping points in chapter 2.

Step 7a. You might start experiencing resistance to tapping and giving up your craving. If this is the case, before you go on to tap on the bright and shiny color, honor the rebel inside and acknowledge the resistance and fear. You can customize the following examples. Remember to check intensity, karate chop while saying the statement one to three times, then tap through the EFT sequence while saying your reminder phrase.

> Even though I question who I will be if I give this up, I accept myself and how I feel.
>
> Even though this is the one thing I know that helps calm me down, I love myself anyway and respect this process.
>
> Even though I'm not giving these up and you can't make me, I completely accept all parts of me, including the younger me who maybe didn't get enough love or attention when she was growing up.

Step 7b. At this point, you might start experiencing some sadness, upset, loneliness, or grief or any other emotion that at one time wasn't okay or safe to feel. You may not know where these feelings come from or which event they may be related to. That's okay, tap on it anyway. Focus on the feeling—it is part of what's holding the craving locked in place. I can't tell you how many people are surprised at how much emotion they feel at some point during these exercises. Again, it's part and parcel of the process—you are allowing these trapped feelings to release, but you have to feel them first.

Step 8. Let's return to "bright and shiny" from step 7. Once you have tapped a few EFT sequences using the reminder phrase, retest your intensity. If the compulsion toward your crave object because they are bright and shiny has gone down to a 2 or below, move on to a different aspect that's enchanting you.

Step 9. You continue this way, performing the EFT basic recipe and tapping down the points on every aspect that comes up relating to your craving until all are neutralized to zero. You'll see some suggestions for amping up the craving and testing for intensity in step 11.

Note: If you feel suddenly flooded with emotion, keep tapping while tuned into the feelings; they *will* pass. When you're tuned in like this, you can let go of the words.

Step 10. At a certain point, some people will clear the body feeling, the feeling of the craving, and then get in touch with a specific memory that happened much earlier in their lives that is where the core disruption happened. This means the memory is linked to the origins of the craving. Maybe Sam, in exploring the origins of his cravings and overeating of salty foods, remembers back to his childhood, when he used to gobble junk food before his parents got home from work. It turns out he had perfectionist parents who expected far too much of him, and he turned to food to comfort and insulate himself against the anxiety he felt when his parents were home. He got approval from doing what was "beyond his means" but at a cost that he still is paying off today. How could he clear this? Look for specific events and apply Tell the Story technique.

Some people won't remember any specific past event, but the intensity of the body sensations and feelings are still happening. In cases like these, the memory may be "implicit," meaning not consciously remembered. You can go ahead and make up an event in this case and tap on aspects just as you would a "real" past event. You are still accessing the core disruption.

Step 11. Maybe you have resolved the feelings. Maybe you just ate the crave object. Okay, we will take a moment to tap on being okay no matter what just happened. Beating yourself up hasn't worked, so how about accepting yourself instead?

> Even though I just ate the thing I want to get rid of and I can't stand it, I deeply and completely accept and forgive myself. (Reminder phrase: "can't stand that I just ate it")
>
> Even though I feel like I failed, I love myself anyway. (Reminder phrase: "feel like a failure")
>
> Even though I feel so much despair and hopelessness because I gave in again, I love, honor, and accept myself, even if I never get over this. (Reminder phrase: "this despair and hopelessness")

After giving in to a craving, this could be a point where a tapalong can allow you an emotional break from the deep stuff—like a wayside rest on the side of a beautiful winding road with an amazing vista in the distance. This is an alternative to Gold Standard EFT. Here you talk through your feelings, whatever comes up. You can customize as you see fit:

Top of head: I ate the whole darn thing, and I feel like such a failure.

Inside eyebrow: I was supposed to get over this, not give in to it.

Outside eye: Will I ever get through this?

Side of eye: I have no self-control.

Under nose: I don't want anyone to know about this. I'm going to keep it a secret. I'm so ashamed.

Chin: What if I never get over this?

Collarbone: I wish I didn't feel this way, but I do. Or maybe it just means the craving is sitting on some pretty big feelings and hurts.

Under arm: Compassion might be more useful here than beating myself up. I already know how to beat myself up. Now, I'm learning self-compassion. How would it feel to just accept what happened and be okay with it?

Second sequence

Top of head: Still, I should be able to get over this. I should. I'm strong enough. I'm good enough. I'm capable enough. Just not about this. And it matters so much to me.

Inside eyebrow: I'm sad that I can't seem to do it.

Side of eye: I'm angry that I can't seem to fix this. I'm mad that the tapping doesn't seem to work ... or maybe it's working too well and bringing up all the big feelings that I didn't even know were under wraps .... Maybe I could give myself some compassion.

Under eye: Compassion? Yeah, right. Here I am tapping to give up the craving, but I gave into it. If feels so disappointing, like I'll never get it right.

Under nose: But I want to make this change. It's hard to feel the feelings that tapping brings up. That's what feels hard. But the feelings are moving through—finally.

Chin: Am I ready to get over it? Do I really want to? Do I really have to? What if I have to make changes I'm not ready to make?

Collarbone: And what if I don't? What if I don't have to do anything till I'm good and ready. Even if I never release this craving, I'm still okay, lovable, worthy, and sometimes even fun and joyful. I'm still a human being who has value and is worthy of love, including self-love.

Under arm: What if I could accept myself just as I am, craving and all? After all, the craving isn't all of me. It's just a habit I learned a long time ago. I'm just unlearning it now.

Top of head: What if I could accept that I ate the (crave object), even when I didn't want to, and it's still okay? Did I learn to walk in a day? Did I learn to talk in a day? I'm just learning a new skill, and I give myself the time I need to feel my feelings and practice. I honor this process and I honor and acknowledge my courage, faith, strength, resilience, and highest self.

Step 12. Back to the main exercise. If you have resolved the feelings, sensations, resistance, thoughts, events, relating to the craving, now draw on all your senses to answer any of these questions that are relevant to your craving to elicit intensity. This is called uncovering hidden aspects. Tap down the intensity on anything that elicits intensity, all the way down to zero, or until you no longer have any desire for the crave object.

- When you put the package in your hand, how much do you want it now on the 0 to 10 scale?
- When you open the package, how much do you want it now?
- When you see the contents of the package, how much do you want it?
- When you smell the contents of the package, how much do you want it?
- When you bring the contents closer to you, how much do you want it?

- When you think that you will not get to have the contents of the package, how much do you want it?
- When you are afraid you'll be deprived or you're worried about what you'll do or who you'll be without access to the contents of the package, how much do you want it?
- What does this crave object represent to you?
- What feelings are associated with the crave object (include positive, negative, shame, and self-judgment feelings)?
- What self-talk is associated with the crave object?
- What specific memories are associated with the crave object?
- What is this crave object protecting you from? What is it making up for in your life?
- Do the feelings under the crave object remind you of any events in your life in which you had similar feelings?
- What specifically does this crave object give you?
- If there were a metaphor for this crave object, what would it be?

Step 13. Ask yourself if you are neutral about the crave object. If so, do the *in situ* test. Put yourself in the situation with the crave object, and tap on anything else that arises until you are fully neutral about the crave object. If you have a donut craving from a specific store, you will be able to go to that store and pass it by without any feeling of wanting. If you do have wanting, tap on that.

Remember to also include tapping for what the object represents to you. Separate the food from the emotion, as I described in Zoe's case earlier. In Zoe's case, the emotional issues under the cravings were positive and comforting. More often, however, the issues are times in a person's life when he or she has felt scared, alone, helpless, or lost. When the craving is salty, ask yourself, what does this salt need represent to me? Rubbing salt in the wound in your life? Sweet cravings? Where do you need more sweetness, kindness, and love in your life? For a cheese craving: Where does it not feel safe to express yourself or be who you are? Where do you feel the need to insulate yourself to protect your vulnerability? How can you give yourself (or a younger version of yourself) what you needed?

Weight Issues and Body Image and Stress

As you probably know by now, losing weight isn't *really* about the weight. As you found out with cravings, it's not the object that's the problem. It's what's under the craving that's driving the craving—undigested emotional drivers keeping the weight on. These types of issues are what may be in the way of accepting yourself with confidence and joy.

What you may not know is that not being able to accept yourself as you are or how you look, can cause stress. If each time you see your reflection you feel horrible about yourself, if each time you're at the gym you're embarrassed and judgmental and jealous, you are creating a stressful situation inside. The mind creates a negative cascade, sending an electrical impulse to every part of your body letting it know you're *stressed out*. It initiates production of the hormone cortisol, which is known to keep weight on a body and is a culprit in many other diseases, including adult-onset diabetes. Cortisol is nicknamed the "weight-gain hormone." If you are consistently telling yourself how bad you look, how fat you are, how hopeless your situation is, that you can't possibly be happy until you achieve your target weight, or similar, you'll be under significant amounts of stress. Every time you think about or look at your body, feel hungry, consider eating, or compare yourself to someone else's body, your body listens—it can't help it! And it will respond (obey your orders) by releasing cortisol.

If this is what happens for you, interrupt the downward spiral by tapping right there on the spot. You can heal! There will be a time in your life when you accept your body—maybe even *love* your body (or at least like it a little bit)—just as it is. (Even though I don't believe her ... it will never happen for me ... I'd sure like to believe it.)

With acceptance, you may still have pain, but your *resistance* to reality is what causes suffering. And as you unearth the emotional drivers under the cravings, the entire issue will collapse.

Exercise: Experimenting with Self-Talk

Does this kind of self-talk about the future sound familiar? *I'll be happy when .... I'll have a good life when .... If I could just lose ____, I'd ....* Ask yourself what you believe to be true about your life because of your weight. For example, *I'll never have the boyfriend, the wedding, the trip, the promotion ... until I lose ____ pounds.* This fantasy ideal may be the thing in your way! Ask yourself, *What if I didn't need to weigh 150/99/250/130/180/ pounds to be happy, have peace, enjoy life, have more fun, dress well, and feel lighter?* Focus on the feeling that question gives you. Find the feeling and tap on it until the weight no longer matters. It's metaphorical weight. You will have found the real feelings, memories, drivers, and roots beneath the weight—and that's something you can tap on. As always, things change when you tap. When the weight no longer matters, who knows what wonders your feelings of self-acceptance will do for your life and body.

Case Study: Rooting Out Memories, Weight and Body Themes, Clearing Guilt

In this story, the experiences of a client named Shelley illustrate the importance of rooting out the early memories around weight, food, and body image and how becoming aware of yours can reduce the stress and anxiety that lead to overeating. When you clear the guilt, shame, blame, and other hurtful feelings, you unlock the reasons you hold on to the weight.

Shelley experienced stress dozens, maybe hundreds of times a day with all of her negative thoughts, beliefs, talk, and feelings about her weight and body. On the outside, it looked like she had everything. She was an intelligent, caring woman in her mid-thirties, a master therapist with a successful career. But she was locked in a world where she bombarded herself with insecurities about her weight and her body. She noted using eating to assuage her feelings of insecurity in relation to just about everyone else in the world. She didn't feel comfortable in her own skin and even stressed out about whether what she was wearing was going to meet the approval of her colleagues. Her fears made no logical sense, but they made emotional sense given her background. An oldest child, while growing up she was the one who always had to "look perfect" and "be the best," and "take care of everyone else" to get approval.

Shelley's goal was to end the horrible haunting she experienced every day, find peace in who she was, feel comfortable in her own body, and lose weight. But before she could do any of that, she needed to lose some of the *emotional* weight and upset that was actually weighing her down in many different areas of her life.

As is common with many individuals dealing with painful weight and body-acceptance challenges, Shelley regularly thought about negative images throughout the day. Whenever she felt stress, anxiety, or upset, she thought about food and eating; whenever she looked in a mirror or store window, she remembered her latest overeating, her lack of control around food cravings, and the number of failed diets she'd had. From there it was easy to unfavorably compare herself to any woman around her age at the gym, a restaurant, or an event. She even began worrying that the waitress would think she was eating too much if she ordered a substantial meal. And because she was also in the National Guard, she would be regularly weighed, so she was on *her* guard with anything weight-related.

Can you see the many specific events or issues under her feelings about her weight? Did you notice how her constant negative self-talk and self-image affected her weight *and* her confidence?

Many things triggered her, but I asked her questions to discover what feelings were underneath the situations that eating helped her assuage. "The feeling that I'm a fake and a fraud," she said. What if people found out? Her answer: "Then they will see me and I'll be left all alone." And then? "And then I'll die alone."

This way of thinking is quite common. If you ask yourself what will happen when the "bad" thing happens, you will likely go down the rabbit hole of being left to die all alone, a horrible death. Regularly start asking yourself about the worst-case scenario if the "bad" thing happens ... and then what ... and what then ... ? You'll inevitably find out that saying no to your pushy sister is somehow equated in your emotional being with being cast out of the tribe and dying in isolation. Again, it's just another way to begin to tap around the edges of old, big hurts and begin clearing them.

We'll continue with Shelley's story after this exercise. Please customize as you see fit.

Exercise: To Take the Edge Off, Start Slow

Let's start with something global: "I don't like the way I look."

Step 1. Pick something specific about the way you look that you don't like: poochy stomach, gray hair, wrinkles, bad teeth, big feet, varicose veins, too short or tall, too fat or skinny, big thighs, a limp, a birthmark, etc.

Step 2. Rate your tapping target's intensity on the 0 to 10 scale.

Step 3. Tap continuously on the Karate Chop point while repeating three times your phrase that captures the tapping target intensity for you, such as: "Even though I don't like the way I look, don't like my poochy stomach, I deeply and completely accept myself."

Step 4. Tap down the points using a reminder phrase that reminds you of the problem, such as: "poochy stomach."

Step 5. After tapping, rate your intensity again. If it's higher than a 2, get even more specific about this one aspect you don't like. Repeat if necessary (meaning your intensity is a 2 or more) before going to the next aspect on your personal list.

Step 6. Tap as already described above with the new aspects one at a time until the intensity subsides on each one. Think of ocean waves that break on the beach and recede.

Step 7. You can go deeper into this exercise by using a mirror and tapping on the intensity that arises when you look at your body. I went from disliking my gray hair to owning my worth as a woman of wisdom. I'm a woman who has lived a full and wonderful life, and I grew my hair out. It's now shoulder length and I love it.

Going Deeper into Weighty Issues

Remember the metaphor idea? Just the word "weight" can be a metaphor for your life. What is weighing you down? What in your life do you find too heavy? What is weighty in your life that you must take very seriously? Now think about the phrase "weight loss." "Loss" signifies something departing, and with loss comes sadness and grief. No wonder we don't want to "lose" our weight! Try replacing the phrase "weight loss" with "weight release." The word "release" connotes freedom and relief; and with that comes joy and happiness.

Here are a few more questions to consider. What do you believe to be true about yourself or the world or life because of this aspect of yourself that you don't like or find upsetting? What proof (events) do you have that this aspect about yourself is true? What's the self-talk now about your weight, body image, or food? Do you feel desperate, hopeless, or other upsetting feelings when you think about the diets you haven't maintained? Do you blame and judge yourself as weak for not achieving your ideal weight? Have you always considered yourself "the fat one" in the family or among your friends? Have you been ashamed of yourself because of your eating habits? Do you keep your feelings about your weight a secret out of fear that people will find out "who you really are"? And try these: What are you insulating yourself from with the weight? What does weight signify for you? Is it insulating you from intimacy? Is it keeping you from being vulnerable? What would happen if you did reach your ideal weight? How would your life change?

Now, you have even more tapping targets, and that means you have a chance to change it all. Tap on what you believe to be true or an event that seems to "prove" that it's true, until you experience relief.

Others have used setup phrases like these as they step around the edges of the issue:

> Even though I'm a hopeless case and will never be the weight I want, I love, honor, and accept myself.
>
> Even though I feel so heavy all the time, I love, honor, and accept myself.
>
> Even though there must be something wrong with me, or otherwise I'd stop eating like this, I love, honor, and accept myself.
>
> Even though I have to be at my ideal weight to have the life I want, I love myself no matter what.

Even though I have so much despair around this, I love, honor, and accept myself.

If you're having resistance to acceptance, remember you can also tap on the tail-enders or "yeah buts" one at a time down to zero. As you do this, specific events may arise. Tap on each of them and they'll start to generalize, so there aren't as many to do as you think.

More on Shelley's Case: Weight Release and Core Issues

Shelley and I tapped on the unhappiness about her body and what it meant to her. I asked her a series of questions to gain more awareness of the history behind her body hatred, weight despair, and negative self-talk patterns as I looked for specific originating events behind her weight and body-confidence challenges.

She despaired when she thought about her weight problems in relationship to others' bodies. "When was the first time you felt that despair feeling?" I asked her.

If she could not remember a specific event, I was prepared to ask her other questions: "When did you first start feeling uncomfortable about your weight?" "What's the earliest memory you have of feeling 'fat,' overweight, ashamed of how you look?" "When did you realize you felt uncomfortable about your body?" "When have you felt like this before? Who was there?" "What kinds of people 'cause' you to feel this way?"

In your own work, be persistent. Even if you don't get answers the first or second or tenth time, you are working *toward* resolving the upsets that are keeping you stuck in this problem.

Shelley's first memory of feeling despair was when she was six years old, walking with a grown-up cousin at a community pool. Both young Shelly and her adult cousin were in bikinis, but Shelley remembered feeling "fat," like the bikini was too small for her. Now she had in her mind a specific picture; just a flash that lasted about ten seconds of the two of them walking. She named the event "Six and Too Fat." The feeling was despair. She guessed it to be about a 4 in intensity.

Shelley and I tapped on this event using Tell the Story, which turned out to have many aspects, including the feeling of being next to the cousin and the color of the bathing suit. She noted an uncomfortable feeling and a feeling of being exposed, being seen. An insight came to mind—it's about being seen, fear of being seen. I said nothing, because I wanted to see what would unfold first.

We tapped on each of the aspects of the event of "Six and Too Fat" using Tell the Story until she had no charge and even had a hard time recalling much detail. It took all of an hour, if that. After tapping, she reported feeling lighter and more at peace regarding her weight.

When next she visited her hometown, she reported back that she had not gone for the junk food at her parents' house nor had she done any other unhealthy eating behaviors. And she had tapped herself "off a cliff" when she started to compare herself to the young, beautiful, and thin waitress.

We worked over the next several months, and she stopped feeling like a fraud. She started feeling good about herself and her life. She let go of a relationship she'd been in because she thought no one else would have her. She became involved in a relationship where she began to experience emotional intimacy for the first time. Rather than feeling like a fraud, she owned the wonderful woman and person she is.

Identifying the Triggers for Overeating, Self-Hatred, Cravings

On the road to body confidence, Shelley identified more triggers that led her to overeating in the first place. If you don't get at the triggers that stimulate overeating, you won't root the problem out at its core—it can always come back. But what if you don't know your triggers? Most people don't, but you can use EFT to flush them out.

Here are some sample setups to practice addressing the problem of not knowing your triggers or patterns of cravings or overeating. Customize them to suit your own unique situation, then perform the EFT basic recipe, remembering to take an intensity rating before and after each tapping round.

> Even though I don't know why I overeat, don't see my own pattern, I deeply and completely accept myself.

> Even though I forget to look for my self-sabotage and don't see things that are obvious to other people, I love, honor, and accept myself.

> Even though there must be a good reason I sabotage myself (and I'm curious—I wonder what it is and I'd like to explore it in depth), I deeply honor and accept myself.

> Even though I have no idea what the triggers for my overeating are and I'm asking myself to recognize the triggers and help myself become more consciously aware of them, I deeply and completely accept myself, all of me!

In Shelley's case, tapping on phrases like these and allowing herself to experience her feelings began to lift a veil. She began to realize there were many times when she was triggered and in a number of areas. These made her feel uncomfortable and out of control, craving and overeating. Here are some we turned up, for example:

- She had to finish the food on everyone's plates. It was almost a compulsion. She literally felt like she had no choice, whether at a restaurant or at home.
- She had to stop at a certain coffee shop and purchase at least two donuts, and from that shop only. Again, she felt as if

she had no choice. She could not drive by—she *had* to have those donuts.

- The minute she stepped in her parents' door, she wanted to eat.
- Just after a stressful test, she'd crave food. At the time, she was studying to get her masters and working full time.

When she came to see me on this particular day, she was horrified, laden with shame and despair. She had just gone out to eat and had ordered a large meal from the menu. She then proceeded to eat leftovers from her friend's meal, too. I was thrilled that she was experiencing the big old pattern because now we had an opportunity to resolve it!

We tapped on this one experience, just using Shelley's own phrases about her humiliation. I asked, "What does this feeling of humiliation remind you of?" An early memory emerged: She was very little, maybe four or five years old, being "affectionately" called "Big Belly" after sneaking into her mother's lunch box and nibbling her sandwich. "Big Belly" was a term of endearment she'd heard almost all of her life, but when she said the words, tears welled up in her eyes. Clearly we were onto something. There was big hurt there, and we'd found tapping gold. The event was about how she gained approval from her parents. We tapped on every aspect we could find, until when she said the words "Big Belly," she could laugh. What she finally realized is that when she did sneak food or eat off her parents' plates, they thought it was cute and showered her with love and affection. She was essentially praised for overeating and sneaking food! Is it any wonder this pattern had been hard to break?

Shelley was able to resolve her issue with being seen just as she was. She had been the oldest of five kids, and her mom expected her to hold it together. She had to act perfect to gain approval, but inside she was afraid that if anyone really saw what a "mess and fraud" she was, she would be abandoned and die all alone. This was obviously a very old, longstanding belief. We addressed this through stories she shared about her growing up with a mother who treated her like a servant and alternately confided in her inappropriately. Is it any wonder that one of the patterns we broke was her need to sneak as much junk food as she could into her mouth before Mom came home?

Exercise: Creating Your Own Weight Release and Body-Confidence List

List "Weight Release and Body Confidence" as your heading in the EFT journal. Set a timer for five minutes and list specific events where you have felt uncomfortable or frustrated about your body image or your weight. Commit to tapping on these one at a time for your own healing of patterns that no longer serve you.

Your work will help you uncover more roots and the origins of body confidence issues, weight challenges, and craving concerns. These often stretch all the way back through a family line. You might say these are inherited belief systems and patterns of distress that you can uncover and resolve. And you are doing the work for future generations, too.

You Are So Much More Than You Know!

How much of our true nature has to do with how big our boobs or pecs are, or how skinny we are? Our culture emphasizes a form of beauty that is neither real nor reflective of who we are as individuals. On our deathbeds, we're not going to regret not looking like that supermodel on the cover of *Vogue*. You may as well forgive yourself in advance for being so hard on yourself—tap on that one—"Even though I've been so hard on myself and will no doubt continue to be because I am only human, I deeply and completely accept myself anyway."

Imagine that, in your glorious life, you don't have to be anything but yourself. Imagine the expansive feeling of relief, of being at peace, of loving your life, just as you are, in control of your choices, no matter what happens around you.

In Conclusion

In this chapter, we explored how you can address weight challenges and trouble with body image as well as how to clear cravings with EFT. Our next chapter addresses tapping while experiencing loss and grief.

Chapter 11

Loss and Grief—Letting Go with EFT

To sort of paraphrase the poet Kahlil Gibran, the depths of sorrow we feel in our heart are equally proportionate to the heights of joy we are capable of feeling, as paradoxical as it seems. It's not that we seek sorrow, loss, and grief; it usually finds its way to us. But to know that grief has a counterpoint can remind us that grief is not all there is in our lives.

We can use EFT to address loss whether of a loved one or a dream or a way of life or even a favorite bracelet. Tapping will not erase your memory of the loved one, the dream, or the object in question. It addresses the excessive grief, the grief of the unresolved earlier losses in life. Past losses seem to light up each time we experience a new one, and it can result in an energy disruption. For a child, it can seem quite typical; perhaps it is as mundane as losing a special toy, a friend moving away, going from being the one who got all the caregivers' attention to now having to share the spotlight with a new sibling.

To activate your body's energy system, go ahead and tap on the tap-down points, the collarbone point, or the gamut or fingertip points while you read.

Life Is Change

We human beings are continually changing and evolving, despite our best efforts to make things stay the same. We like knowing what to expect because we have a mistaken understanding that the status quo will keep us safe. We don't like losing stuff, but life is about change and letting go.

We leave the sanctity of the womb and are born. We leave our caregiver's arms and begin crawling, walking, and playing independently. We leave the sweet simplicity of childhood and enter into awkward, ungainly, tumultuous, independent adolescence. We leave home, go to college, have careers, marry, and have lives of our own. We watch our children grow...and leave. Our bodies change. Finally, we reach the end of life—another change. Truly, from the moment we are born, "letting go," "leaving behind," and "change" are the operative words. And yet we are often caught off-guard and unprepared with regard to our losses.

When we meet the changes, life works. But when we're burdened by grief, our ability to experience life's wonder and joy is affected. When the feelings get stuck inside, we ourselves get stuck. We displace. We project. We ignore. We do all kinds of creative things to avoid feeling the grief.

Exercise: Releasing Intensity Charge Around the Loss

Here we will gently work with grief you are ready to release.

Step 1. In your EFT journal, create the heading: "Grief and Loss Release." Identify a loss you'd like to work with. It could be anything from loss of a loved one to an experience you believe you have an unreasonable attachment to or would like to experience peace rather than pain.

Step 2. List your thoughts, feelings, sensations, self talk, the details you recall when you think of that loss, or of letting go of grief. Here are examples from my practice from clients who have lost loved ones in all manner of circumstances: "It's not fair." "It's wrong." "There was no closure." "It's unacceptable." "I can't go on now." "Someone needs to pay for this. I'm so angry!" "I am guilty.""I didn't do enough. I should have been there." "It's my fault." "No one understands what it's like." "My life is over." "I feel the loss of what I never had." "The heavy pressure in my chest." "I am suddenly exhausted in my body." "How do I go on after having cared for him/her (who was sick) all these years?" "I just miss her so much." "I feel so alone and unlovable."

Now choose just *one aspect* from your list—this will be the start of your manageable tapping. Simultaneously, note how you feel this aspect inside your body in your journal.

Step 3. Now what's the intensity, 0 to 10, about that aspect you chose? Write it down. You're already aware of your body sensation, as you noted it in step 2.

Step 4. Apply the EFT basic recipe to your tapping target. In this case, we will simply tap on the "top level" of the grief, with this example: "I don't think I can ever get over this." As always, tap on your Karate Chop point one to three times while repeating this setup statement:

> Even though I'll never get over this, I deeply and completely accept myself.

Tap through at least one or more EFT sequences, starting at the top of the head through under the arm, with: "I'll never get over this,"until you sense a shift in intensity.

Step 5. Now take a deep breath, allowing the breath to flow up from the earth, into the soles of your feet, up through your legs, through your torso, and through the crown of your head. Exhale, letting go, with the exhale longer than your inhale. Repeat several times.

Step 6. Check your intensity now on "I'll never get over this." If it is higher, go to step 9. If lower, go to step 8. If it's the same, go to step 7. If your aspect (for example, "I'll never get over this") has subsided and now other aspects of the loss are popping their heads up at sixes and sevens or higher, just allow for their passing, one at a time, EFT round by EFT round. When you get to this step again, keep following through until you experience relief, meaning that you are able to think of the tapping target with neutrality. Or, you are able to think of the person or the event and have more perspective than at the time of loss, for example.

Step 7. If intensity is the same. Do you believe logically that you can never get over this? Do you believe emotionally that you can never get over this? Get more specific. Is it too big? Is it that you don't know how (yet) to navigate this unknown territory? Is it because you never expected it to be this way? Choose one reason you can never get over this. We're getting more specific to get results. Tap with a more specific "I can't get over this because ... " in mind, and see if it doesn't loosen "I can't get over this." Or focus on your body sensations about never getting over this and tap around following a body sensation relating to "never get over this" using Chase the Pain. Or go to an earlier loss, and tap on one event related to that. Then move on to step 10.

Step 8. If intensity is lower. Choose a thought, phrase, feeling, or body sensation that happens when you think of the loss you have identified from step 1, such as: "I am so angry about what happened. It's not fair. It's ...." Skip to step 10 when you are neutral or close to it here. As well, uncover specific events by asking: What about it isn't fair? You may have a laundry list of tapping targets by asking this question. Write them down to tap on now, one at a time before moving on.

Step 9. If intensity is higher. Keep on tapping on the same target you had in step 2. Allow yourself to take a few deep breaths, inhaling all the way from the soles of your feet up through the top of your head, and then out. Again, inhale deeply now through the top of your head, down and out through the soles of your feet. Repeat the process a few more times. Now tune into both your tapping target and your body sensation. Start another round. Here are possible setup statements to inspire you:

> Even though I can't get over this, I love, honor, and accept myself.
>
> Even though a part of me believes I can't get over this, I deeply and completely accept all parts of me.
>
> Even though I can't see how I'll get over this, I accept myself and how I feel right now.

Focus in on your body sensations, and follow them. Allow yourself to cry, or feel the feelings, and keep on tapping through the flood of emotions!

Step 10. Retest your intensity. How much can't you "get over this" now? Or how much is it not fair? Using the tapping example of "can't get over this," ask yourself these questions:

How come I can't get over this? Answer: It's my fault.

How is it my fault? Answer: I wasn't there for him at a critical moment.

How so? Answer: When he was in the hospital that one time, I needed to go home and rest, but he was in pain.

Aha! A specific event underneath one of the many reasons why you "can't get over this." Tap on this with Tell the Story until intensity around this particular event subsides.

Step 11: Now, return to your original tapping target from step 2, here it's "I can't get over this." Now how much do you still believe, or what's left relating to "can't get over this" or whatever tapping target you chose? Do you see how you can begin to see some hope? Even if you have shifted one point, that's movement!

Support for Getting through Grief

In some cultures, the community engulfs the mourner. I don't mean they share their condolences by delivering homemade food or sending cards. The community sits with the mourners until they experience a breakthrough. If we were held through our grief with nothing expected, the experience would be profound and healing for all involved. Consider tapping when you're troubled by these issues: "Even though I need more than what I'm getting right now, I love myself anyway" or "Even though I'm expected to be normal, and how is that even possible right now, I love myself anyway" or "Even though I don't have the support I need through this troubled time . . . ."

An alternative to traditional EFT is to tap continuously while expressing phrases like these until you experience some relief: "It's possible for me to release this grief, according to my own timing." "I know this is hard. And I can still do it." "I am going through the hard stuff now and I'm okay." "It feels like my world is ending, but I'm still here. And I have more resources than I can possibly imagine right now." "I forgive myself for being scared. I forgive myself for hurting. I forgive myself for lashing out. I forgive myself for shutting down. I forgive myself for blaming. I forgive myself for everything I did do, and for everything I didn't do . . . ." "I choose to love, honor, and accept myself." "I shower myself with compassion and kindness." "I am open to healing, to my own wholeheartedness, to myself and to all that is divine in my life." "I feel the soles of my feet on the floor. I feel the earth rising up to meet me." "I choose to breathe in life, and to release everything I no longer need or that is no longer serving me."

Exercise: Releasing Learned Helplessness and Burden

Grief can bring up fear and helplessness about everything you don't know how to do. You may wonder how to go on without the person in your life, how to do the financial statements, to parent on your own, to cook . . . . You may be afraid of future losses. Add the word "yet" to what you don't know how to do in your setup statements. "Yet" gives hope that you can figure it out. It's an alternative to the helplessness or hopelessness you might feel about your loss.

> I don't know how to go on without this person in my life, yet. . . .
>
> I have no idea how to run the business, be a single parent, or cook a decent meal, yet I'm open to learning. I have learned other things, so it's possible I can learn this, too. I am a resilient, capable, resourceful human being.

Step 1. Notice how you are feeling in your body. Make note of any tensions or aches or pains before you get started. Now, aim one EFT round at what you can't do or don't think you can learn how to do.

Step 2. Now, try that same round, adding "yet" to what you don't know how to do.

Even though I have no idea how to do X *yet*, I deeply and completely accept myself.

Step 3. Remind yourself of the many things you had no idea how to do or that you thought were impossible but you ended up doing. Tap all the tap-down points, a single point, or the finger points as you list them aloud. What does it feel like in your body to acknowledge the capacity to grow and change? You are reminding your system that you do, indeed, know how to learn and even now are in the process of learning how to do—even this, even this.

Step 4. Now how do you feel about learning or about the grief target? See if there has been any corresponding change in how you feel in your body.

Case Study: Loss and Grief Shrunk Sima's World

Sometimes a person's world gets really small around the grief object or person. The whole world can seem to revolve around the brief time of the loss, which is just one snapshot in time rather than your whole experience over the course of many years with that person, place, or job.

Sima and her husband had many good times during their fifteen years together. At the time her husband, Robert, contracted an incurable, painful cancer, they had just moved to the land of their dreams, where they had big plans for their careers. The illness was swift. Within months, Robert was gone. Every time Sima thought of him, it was about the brief time in their lives when he was dying. She had no access to the wonderful memories. She felt like she should have done more, especially at key moments in his decline and treatment. She had many specific events holding this belief up. If only she had done something differently, he might have survived. She understood this belief wasn't logical—that it was emotional.

Sima was working with me about being stuck in her job. However, the story of her husband came up in our second session, and she cried as if the loss had been yesterday. She had hundreds of stories about how awful it was, how she wasn't there for him (she had been), and more. We tapped on several of the biggest of the traumatic events till she experienced neutrality. Soon thereafter, she understood that she was staying in the job she'd had since shortly after he died because she was working with people in similar situations to what hers and her husbands' had been. But she was ready to move on now. She no longer equated moving (which they had done right before the cancer was diagnosed) with his suffering, her "inability" to help him, and all the difficult moments surrounding his illness.

Let Grief Out and Resolve It

Unresolved grief is like unrequited love. It can lead to getting stuck in dead-end jobs and shutting down in a marriage. It can give rise to displaced emotions, such as getting overly angry with others or overly angry with ourselves, even though they've/we've done nothing to deserve our wrath. Unresolved grief can lead to depression, difficulty making changes, hoarding, problems with intimacy, and illness. It can mask our joy.

Over time, unresolved grief compounds. Grief from past emotionally unresolved losses has a way of surfacing every time a new loss is experienced.

Additionally, the way we normalize or cope with a loss can sometimes make it difficult for us to experience life to its fullest. Kara had a sister who had been murdered decades back. When Kara went anywhere new, she felt an immediate need to call at least one family member to let them know she was safe. EFT helped her realize there was not a murderer lurking behind every café's door. In another case, Serena's mother had been murdered by her father. Decades later, Serena feared telling her husband the truth about anything she thought might upset him, because she feared he would kill her. After addressing some of the key events with Tell the Story around that belief, she was able to start telling him the truth. The marriage improved and so did her life.

Grief manifests in many ways, from being stuck, body symptoms, and big fears, to self-sabotage of all kinds. Underneath the symptoms are specific events associated with grief. These hold the energy disruption in place. Each event can be tapped with Gold Standard EFT until the whole grief tabletop collapses. Here are some events different clients associated with loss:

- Seeing Mom's face at the funeral
- When I heard the news on the phone
- Not being able to say goodbye
- All the things that couldn't happen with this person
- The last words between us were angry
- What I miss about him
- The punched-in-stomach feeling
- Proof I took him for granted
- What I can't ever tell him now
- Can't talk about him without crying
- What that well-meaning neighbor lady said that really hurt
- What I'd really like to say to some of the well-meaning people in my life who are just making it worse

Remember to note where you are feeling the events in your body as you tap. Keep tapping on your tap-down points while you read.

Secondary Gains and Limiting Beliefs of Grief

Ask yourself what "secondary" gains you are receiving for holding on to the grief. What does your grief give you the excuse to do or not do? How is that affecting your whole life? Grief manifests in some very interesting ways, as you know. List what you are "getting" and tap on your unwillingness to give it up.

Limiting beliefs, core issues, and self-talk surround people dealing with unresolved grief. Many say things they really don't mean, such as "my life is over," or "I'll never recover." You'll want to undo those vows. What vows did you make at the time of your loss? What did you tell yourself? What decisions did you make? What do you believe about yourself as a result of the loss? These are generally not beneficial vows, decisions, self-talk, and beliefs. How are these things playing out in your life? Simply becoming aware of these decisions is the beginning of releasing them.

Case Study: Dawn's Loss Stopped Her in Her Tracks

When Dawn learned her sister had died, she said "my life is over," and "it's my fault." She acted like it too. Nothing moved for her after the death some five years back. She no longer traveled, exercised, was stuck in a dead-end job, and was tired all the time. "How could I not have been there for her?" she thought often. We started with what she missed about her sister, what she didn't get to do with her sister, and then she was able to start to share some of the good times she and her sister had. We tapped on her sadness that those good times were over—until she realized she could touch upon them any time in her mind and experience the joy. Finally, we went to the day it happened, tapping on the knock on the door, the police officer's face, the way she knew, where her brother was standing, the thoughts that came to mind, the belief that her life was over, the belief that it was her fault, the guilt, and more until she had neutrality here.

We "undid" the vow she had made, and her belief that life was over changed—a shift in belief. Dawn understood her sister's death was not her fault; she had done everything she could, and she could not have prevented it (this is the cognitive shift). She had more energy in her daily life and her vitality returned. (This is what emotional release can feel like.) She made travel plans, began to exercise again, created and began circulating a new resume. She signed up for a week-long "change-maker" workshop, and her fear of losing her job because she was wrong had all but dissipated. (These are behavioral shifts.) Life again had possibility.

Case Study: Jean's Underground Grief and Her Seemingly Unrelated Problems

Jean couldn't say her mother's name without crying, even five years after the death. She was having difficulty parenting and was especially resentful of her youngest child. There were problems in her marriage (especially relating to her husband "being there" for her), low self-esteem causing trouble for her at work, and an intense phobia of germs. A vibrant full-time working mother of two young children, Jean had shut down so she could at least function, but she was a prisoner to her loss. Grief had robbed her of her ability to see the whole.

After tapping, the specific event that came up was the time when Jean was eight months pregnant with her youngest, exhausted, and visiting her dying mother. Key aspects included her mother hadn't been there emotionally for her (she was dying), the mom said bad things about Jean's toddler, and her husband hadn't been able to come with her on this visit. We tapped on all aspects we could uncover until Jean was neutral and reported feeling much lighter. Another session involved tapping on everything she didn't get from her mom at that crucial time when she was pregnant, and everything she couldn't do for her mom because she was pregnant and working full time. Over the next several sessions, Jean reported that she was no longer tearing up at her mom's name or resentful of her youngest. She understood she'd projected the lack of being there from her mom onto her husband, and her marriage began to improve. She began sleeping better, and the germ phobia (which had been related to an aspect of her mom's illness) disappeared. She experienced more joy in all areas of her life, especially with her children.

Questions Relating to a Loss in Your Life

Think about what you have told yourself, what decisions you have made, and what beliefs you have formed about yourself or the world as a result of your loss. Do you have unresolved fears about making changes or about losing someone or something? What happens when you think of giving up what you no longer need? Do you want to make the change but feel as though something's holding you back? What might that be, if you had to guess? What happened the last time you made a big change? What is your earliest memory of loss? Did anyone help you understand the loss? If there are stories about it that you don't remember because you were too young, what are the key points of the story? Has that loss affected you, and if so, how? Are there areas of your life where it still hurts to think of a part of your life that is now long over, or to think of something or someone or a dream that has long since died?

Little Losses and Letting Go

You don't even have to have big, capital-T Trauma to have unresolved grief. What I'm talking about are little losses growing up. What happened when you lost something growing up? Children feel keenly—have you ever seen a tantrum? Maybe you lost the full attention of your parents when your younger sibling was born? What happened when your caregivers experienced loss? How was it handled or not handled in your family? As a child, when you expressed grief and sadness about a loss, what happened in your family? If your primary caregivers weren't comfortable with grief, you might associate that particular feeling with emotional abandonment. You can uncover the specific tappable events when you look back.

When we experience the fullness of weaning, it means we have dealt with our feelings relating to the letting go. Then we can make the shift, process the emotions around it, and move on. If we learned that letting go and moving on is scary, we may have trouble finishing cycles, whether that means leaving one job for a more fulfilling one, letting go of an unhealthy friendship, or grieving the loss of a loved one and moving on.

As you tap, allow yourself to have and experience the grief of the loss now. The waves will rise, then recede. Once you have reached neutrality on an event, notice what changes. Notice any changes in your body. Notice if the way you are thinking or acting in another area of your life has changed. Write these changes down so you remember them for the next time.

Exercise: Releasing Unresolved Early Feelings of Grief

What weanings were not fully resolved in your own life? Write them down. Then, tap on the specific incidents, one at a time, one aspect at a time.

You may need to tap on everything you are angry, sad, etc., about *before* you get to the forgiveness part. Rose's husband had died and left her in a very bad financial situation with three young children. She had suffered chronic pain for many years now. As she began addressing her pain, up came feelings and memories about the loss of her husband some thirty years back. She first needed to neutralize the feelings of abandonment, anger, helplessness, fear, sadness, and more. She tapped on specific events relating to the time of the loss before she was able to forgive her husband and feel at peace. As a bonus, the chronic pain eased once she released those negative feelings.

Following are some examples of general tapping setup statements you can customize:

Sadness, anger, loneliness, or hopelessness: "Even though I'm (hurting) about the loss, I am still here and okay." (Reminder phrase: "hurting about this grief")

Resistance: "Even though I'll never get over this and my life is over...."(Reminder phrase: "never get over it")

Feeling alone: "Even though I'm all alone in this and may be for the rest of my life, I deeply and completely accept myself anyway." (Reminder phrase: "I'm all alone")

Avoiding grief: "Even though I can't bring myself to think about (this grief), it's not bigger than I am, and I am safe." (Reminder phrase: "cannot think about this grief")

Afraid: "Even though just thinking about (this grief) is scary, I bless these feelings, and it is my intention to heal." (Reminder phrase: "it's too scary")

Letting go: "Even though I want to hold on to (this grief) because it's all I have left, it is possible there's more to remember that will bring me joy." (Reminder phrase: "want to hold on to this")

Feeling helpless/like a victim: "Even though it feels like I have no control over (this grief), I am open to the possibility that I can make different choices and release some of the extra grief." (Reminder phrase: "cannot control this")

Heavy feeling in body: "Even though I feel this heavy grief feeling in my body (name where, if you can sense it), I deeply and profoundly accept all of my feelings and am grateful to my body for showing me where I'm storing it." (Reminder phrase: "I feel it in my body here")

Reason to keep the grief: "Even though it would be a betrayal to get over (this grief), I deeply and profoundly accept myself." (Reminder phrase: "it's wrong to get over this")

Guilt over the grief: "Even though it's my fault, and you are not going to convince me otherwise, even God makes mistakes. I wonder if it's possible to forgive myself." (Reminder phrase: "it's all my fault")

Angry over the loss: "Even though I'm still angry and will never forgive them about what happened, I deeply and profoundly accept all my feelings and would prefer to release the anger keeping me prisoner." (Reminder phrase: "I'm really angry and will never forgive them")

Angry at person: "Even though I'm really mad at you for what you did, I accept myself, I accept you, and I want to see this differently today." (Reminder phrase: "mad at ___")

Exercise: Grief List for EFT Journal—A Plan of Action

Try the Personal Peace Procedure. List your losses and tap on them one at a time. Examples may span from loss of first tooth to not making varsity to losing that relationship to the time we moved to the divorce, and so on. It may help to start with the small stuff. Remember that when you work on one target, you're effectively working on all events under that tabletop or in that spiral. And as you know by now, a generalization effect will kick in at a certain point.

Determine Aspects of Each Specific Grief Incident

The following questions are designed to elicit aspects for you to tap on relating to your tapping targets.

- When did the grief incident happen?
- If there were a place in your body you were storing the grief incident, where would it be? Is there an awareness of a certain body part when you think of the incident?
- Is there a color, flavor, smell, image, texture, weight, or other quality you associate with the grief incident?
- Who was there with you when you experienced the grief incident?
- Do you wonder what you would do without this particular incident?
- How does feeling this affect you in your daily life? If you're not sure, guess.
- How will it feel to let it go? Is it safe to let it go? What's preventing you from moving on?

- How would your life change if you were free of this grief from the incident?
- What story are you telling yourself about the grief incident?

What If I Believe It's Too Much to Handle?

When you feel like the grief is locked in hard and won't budge, consider it as the outermost ring of the tree. The stuckness you're experiencing is a symptom of the feelings underneath. Try tackling the resistance around the edges. You might want to tap taking inspiration from these possible setups:

> Even though this grief is just never going to go away, there may come a time when I'm ready to let it go, just not quite yet.
>
> Even though it feels like my life is over only if I choose to let it be, I may change my mind about this later.
>
> Even though I can't stand what happened, there may be a time when I can accept it as reality.
>
> Even though I can't relate to people anymore, maybe I can again someday.
>
> Even though I don't want to do this, not wanting to do this doesn't mean I am not capable of it when I am ready.
>
> Even though this grief is not going to budge, it might shrink.
>
> Even though this is too much to deal with and I won't and don't ever have to if I don't want to, I remember a time when I was okay.

If you grew up in a family where it wasn't okay to express feelings of sadness, you may want to tap on issues like: "I'm not allowed to grieve," "it's not okay to feel sad," "what's wrong with me that I'm still upset?" "Part of me has been holding on to the sadness I had no one to share with when I was so little," "I can't express my hurt because they don't like it."

Case Study: Early Loss Explains Dan's Roots of Anxiety and Insomnia

Dan's father died when Dan was three. Now in college, Dan had anxiety, difficulty concentrating, and wouldn't go to sleep except late into the night, which perpetuated the cycle. These were the symptoms of the problem, but not the problem itself. As we tapped about his anxiety, I asked him the famous question: "What does this remind you of?" The loss of his father came to mind. We tapped on specific incidents around this early loss, including: waking up to the news at age three and not understanding why Dad wasn't coming back and a time at the playground where he was having fun and then looked at his mother and realized that he should not be having fun but instead act sad.

Among other interesting insights, Dan's unconscious belief causing the insomnia he had suffered for many years bubbled to the surface. In his young life, he had refused to go to sleep unless completely exhausted. Finally, we got to the core. The limiting belief was: "If I fall asleep, someone I love will die." Dan had been asleep when his father died. In the three-year-old worldview of his subconscious, no one would die if he stayed awake.

He also had a knee-jerk reaction to be overly kind and caring to people when saying goodbye, even if they were near strangers or he didn't like them. The underlying belief here was: "I need to be nice and say goodbye because otherwise they might die." He had not had a chance to say goodbye to his father. He worked through his unresolved grief from so long ago. His anxiety decreased significantly. His "goodbye" compulsion ended, and he no longer had problems saying goodbye. He completed college free of insomnia and went onto a wonderful teaching career.

Letting Go of Dreams

Letting go of what you dreamed you would have but that never happened is a form of grieving, too. If being married is your dream and it doesn't seem to be happening, you may have grief to tap on. If you are divorcing, you may have the grief of not spending your lives together and everything that meant to you. There's grief over the loss of health or over aging. There's grief over not being able to have your own biological baby if that has been your expectation and your identity has been wrapped up in it. The tapping might extend in this case to events like how painful it is to be around pregnant women or to listen to colleagues at work discuss their children. Once you collapse the grief around lost dreams, you'll find it's much easier to open up to new ones.

In Conclusion

We've explored how you can begin to poke around the edges of grief and loss, as well as how to use EFT to gently release and navigate through the small and big losses in your life.

You now have a sound foundation from which to continue your tapping practice. You've learned one-point tapping and Gold Standard EFT. You've tried the exercises and gotten results. You've probably been surprised a time or two at how quickly tapping works. And you've likely shared tapping with a friend, or ten.

You know you can tap any time, anywhere, and on anything. You know EFT terminology and how to look under your big tabletop issues to uncover the specific events holding a problem in place. You know how to aim EFT at one event at a time, tapping on one aspect at a time, until the whole event collapses. You know that if you tap enough events through to neutrality, the whole issue will collapse and you'll experience relief.

You've built on the basics to include Tell the Story technique, which gives you a system to dismantle the charge from bad memories step by step. You've learned how to resolve physical symptoms and uncover emotional contributors to pain through Chasing the Pain. And you know how to begin to use EFT to address a broad spectrum of challenges, including changing unhealthy life-stress patterns, resolving self-sabotage, clearing cravings, restoring body confidence, addressing excess unresolved grief, ending phobias, clearing the emotional contributors to physical illness, obtaining pain relief, and more.

As you continue to grow in your practice you'll continue to experience wow! moments as longtime issues dissolve with as few as one round of tapping. You also know that to get results, you have to be persistent! May this book be a resource for you time and again.

Appendix A
Tapping Summary

EFT basic recipe

1. Identify a tapping target—a troubling feeling, sensation, thought, or bad memory.
2. Rate the current intensity of the issue on the 0 to 10 scale. Zero is completely neutral, 10 is the most intense.
3. Insert the tapping target into the EFT template to create the EFT setup statement.
4. Express the EFT setup statement one or more times while continuously tapping the Karate Chop point.
5. Create an EFT reminder phrase, shorthand for the tapping target.
6. Tap the eight points of the EFT tapping sequence while repeating the reminder phrase, start top of head to under arm.
7. Test the 0 to 10 intensity number again after tapping one or two sequence rounds.
8. Adjust for changes in intensity by tweaking your setup phrase or creating a different setup phrase, and start the process all over again until all references to the upset are wholly dissolved

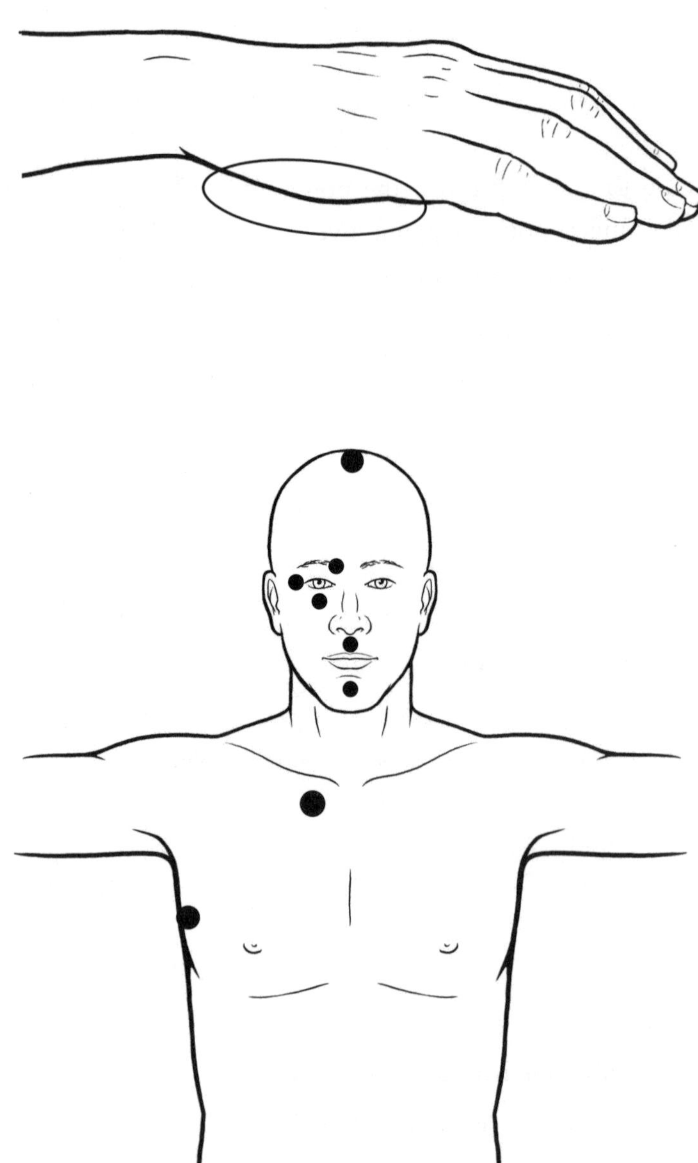

Figure 6: The Karate Chop point (top); the EFT sequence (bottom)

Additional Tapping Points

Fingertip Points

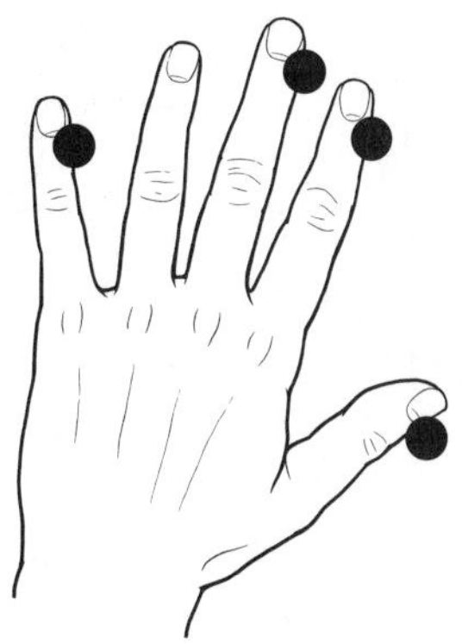

After performing the EFT basic recipe, including the tapping down the points, you add finger points tapping five to seven times on each point below:

- Outside humb at base of nail
- Inside index finger
- Inside middle finger
- Inside baby finger
- Karate Chop point

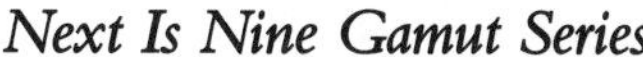

Next Is Nine Gamut Series

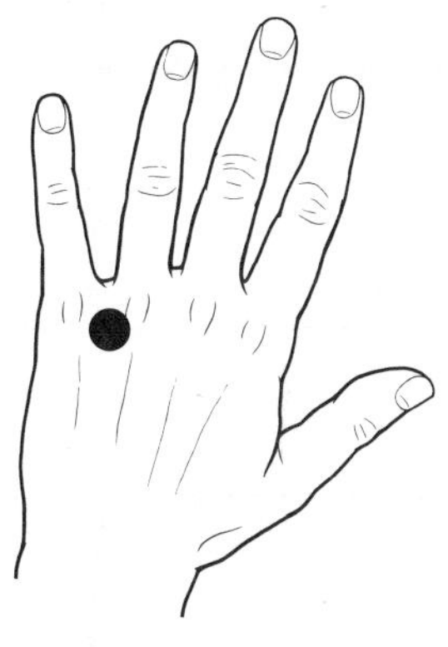

Locate the gamut point between the ring and pinkie fingers, about one inch back from the knuckles. Tap this point gently and continuously through the nine-gamut series. Holding the associated problem in your mind:

1. Close your eyes.
2. Open your eyes.
3. Eyes only, look hard down to the right.
4. Eyes only, look hard down to the left.
5. Move your eyes clockwise a full circle.
6. Move your eyes counterclockwise in a full circle.
7. Hum two seconds of a song.
8. Count rapidly from 1 to 5.
9. Hum two seconds of a song again.

Repeat the EFT sequence.

You can start with the EFT basic recipe, continue with tapping fingers, the gamut points, and one more EFT sequence as a full round. Do it as one whole flow.

Below Nipple Point or Liver Point

Located one inch below the nipple on a male, and where the breast attaches to the chest for a female. It's not as easy to access especially in public, but it's very useful.

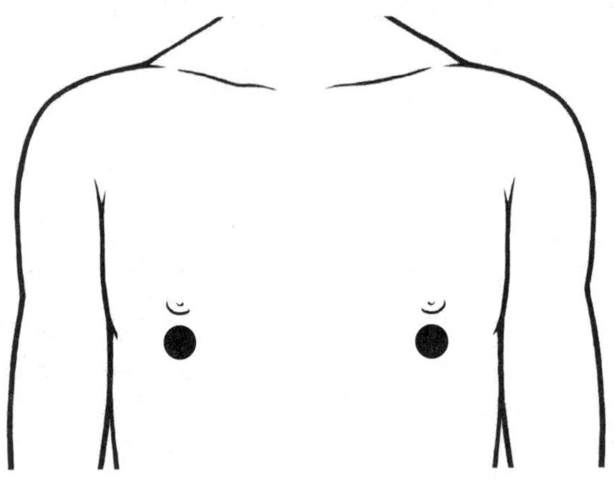

Wrist Points

You can tap the wrist point of each hand either with fingertips or by just tapping both wrists together.

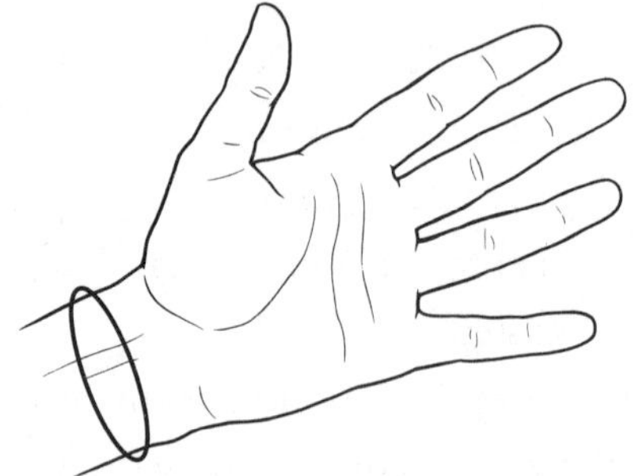

Appendix B
Taking a Wayside Rest from the Tough Stuff

Is it time for a wayside rest? Do you need to take the edge off all this serious stuff we are talking about and try a positive tapping exercise? Here are a few ways you can take a break from the serious stuff when you need to step away.

Wayside Rest 1

Note these taps offer the equivalent of an emotional wayside rest when you need it. They are a variation of traditional EFT. Let's have a quick restorative moment.

Step 1. First, breathe deeply for a count of four, double your exhale to a count of eight. Repeat four times before going to the next step.

Step 2. Tap on your thymus/collarbone points while expressing these words or any phrases that give you a good feeling:

"Isn't life grand? I'm learning how to tap. I'm learning a lot about myself. It's possible to heal, and I'm healing now. I love the idea of feeling better. I love feeling good. I love sunrises. I love the colors of the sunset. I love the sound of the crickets on a midsummer's night. I love the sound of my favorite song. I love the song of my soul."

Good! We can move on now. Feel free to take a wayside rest like this any time you're feeling even a little overwhelmed as you read through the book.

Wayside Rest 2

It's useful to know that we can dip in and out of big feelings and that they are not the boss of us, so to speak. What were your favorite upbeat songs growing up? Compile a list and then access that music in a playlist. Listen to it, sing it, play it, dance it, enjoy it now. Play it when you need a "now for something completely different" moment.

The resting space can allow you the space to remember that the troubling event is not all of you and will not swallow you up. These rests serve as reminders of what a wonderful and amazing human being you are just as you are right now, problems and all.

Wayside Rest 3

How do you feel right now? Tap your finger points or the tap-down points while reliving a super positive event that happened in the past. Be specific and relive the wonderful details about that good experience. Savor it. Juice it. Now notice if your mood has changed. If you're ready, go back now to your tapping target, equipped with the most effective tool in the universe: an open heart.

Appendix C
EFT Resources

Here's information directly and indirectly related to tapping or healing I've found helpful. This is not a comprehensive resource section, just a selection of items you may find useful or that I have enjoyed. Websites evolve quickly, so some may no longer be available.

Tapping Variations and the Evolution of Energy Therapy

When EFT was developed by Gary Craig in 1995, his open-handed, generous approach, coupled with the technique being so easy and profoundly effective, helped spread meridian therapy throughout the world. An online newsletter that began with twenty people fairly rapidly had some 500,000 subscribers. Workshops were attended by hundreds, but there was not one-on-one teaching in these venues. The standards of EFT and even what constitutes EFT has come to vary widely, and like any innovation, is an ongoing topic of discussion and controversy. Some people learned EFT at the workshops, others from DVDs, others by watching a YouTube video, still others from someone who had attended a workshop. The approach, experience, instruction, standards, intent, and applications of practitioners and tapping trainers have varied widely. What constitutes EFT is regularly under question. And that is a good thing, because as we clarify what works safely with individuals in need, the whole field improves. However, the field can occasionally be likened a bit to the Wild West. Gary Craig has noted that he believes he made a "blunder" when initially introducing EFT in a way that opened its use to the world when the practice lacked a standardized way to consistently teach and monitor those who were teaching as well as the practitioners being certified. In recent years, he and his daughter, Tina Craig, implemented clear, consistent standardized teaching methods and standards for EFT: Gold Standard EFT. Their well-thought-out, thorough, and comprehensive tutorials with guided, step-by-step information, will enhance your practice and ability to get results. Gary Craig's emofree.com is the no cost teaching site of which I am a member and which I frequently revisit to refine my own technique. The site now also includes his latest development and exploration into healing, which explores in essence, the spiritual nature of healing and its practical applications.

EFT Credentials: A Brief History

Early on, tests were administered through EFT founding master Pat Carrington, PhD, and author of the Choices Method of EFT. Those who passed the tests received a certificate of completion of a test: EFT Level 1 and EFT Advanced. Next came the more rigorous earning of credentials EFT Certification (Cert)-1, II, and Honors. These required that you had a practice and understood and were extensively versed in the concepts and the tapping techniques. Prior to the onset of these programs, there was a program for advanced EFT practitioners—EFT Masters Program (and all masters are considered Honors practitioners), which required significant commitment and admission on a one-on-one basis. That program, begun in approximately 2005, came to an end in 2007, with just twenty-nine Masters having completed it.

In the ensuing years, Tina Craig developed and directed the Gold Standard EFT ACP-EFT and ACEP-EFT credentialing system through the Association for Comprehensive Energy Psychology (ACEP), an organization that also includes licensed therapists and other mental health and holistic practice professionals. In my experience earning the ACP-EFT credential, this is the most comprehensive, extensive, and thorough program in the use of Gold Standard EFT. It included extensive one-on-one mentoring, significant video session review with detailed feedback of each technique in the EFT toolkit, and required mastery at a very high level. The program has made me a more thorough, effective professional and my sessions have become more powerful with regard to results. As of this writing, Tina Craig is stepping down as director in December 2015. Training continues, however.

Another solid program for earning excellent credentials, in my experience, is the Association for Advancement of Meridian Techniques (AAMET) International, with four practitioner levels. It features excellent training and generous insightful mentoring by the knowledgeable, capable, and thorough Jondi Whitis.

Should you wish to pursue professional aspirations as a practitioner, add it into your clinical practice, or just learn more about the technique, there are Level 1 and Level 2 trainings, as well as trainings otherwise designated that provide excellent training. It pays to research, whether the individual practitioner is working under the banner of a designated organization or on his or her own. Some excellent teachers do not teach under any organizational banner, for example. Obtain personal referrals about the trainer. Speak one on one to those who attended a past seminar or training. Consult with the trainer to gain an understanding if this is a good fit for you. Note also that the size of an organization does not necessarily denote teaching quality. Some practitioner trainers teach under one of the above-named organization's banners. Others teach under

EFTUniverse, and still others teach as mentioned not under any banner, and yet others teach their own brand of EFT. Research the trainer's bona fides, and go beyond the testimonials—anyone can write a testimonial.

Other Tapping Methods

As noted, Gold Standard is not the only meridian tapping that gets results. Others who have developed their own approaches concurrent with the development with EFT also are effective. Many early energy tapping pioneers as well as the early adopters of EFT who initially learned from Gary Craig have created their own protocols, even their own brands of tapping. The issue is not variations, in my opinion—because I am a personal recipient of variations working. There are many, many ways to scale a mountain, and all roads as is said, lead to home, as opposed to Rome. To me, the problem arises when practitioners have not done their own inner work and do not have the knowledge, the wisdom, the healthy boundaries, or the clarity inside, to help people clear issues out at the roots, whatever their approach, or do not know or are even aware of how to work ethically and safely with people, especially those who have experienced Trauma with a capital T. Such people may not be aware or responsive to the issues tapping can raise. Some individuals with unresolved significant mental health issues or those who aren't aware of the big stuff they've been sitting can find themselves drowning when they follow along with a workshop leader or online practitioner who isn't taking all of this into account.

Tapping is powerful. To me, it works with body, mind, and spirit, and that includes the electromagnetic energy system of the body. When you are working with deep stuff, you want someone who not only knows how to swim in the deep waters but also able and adept at bringing you easily and gently back to shore repeatedly, so you can finally do it independently after some practice. Remember that you and your money can be easy pickings when you're feeling desperate and believe the answers are outside of you. The wizards of Oz behind the curtain exist in every emerging field.

Gold Standard techniques are the centerpiece of my EFT practice. And there are other holistic methods that I have drawn on in my healing work that may include tapping variations, the use of song, music-making, writing and other creative arts, body movement, and body shaking and trembling to release trauma, deep listening, herbal consultations, health coaching sessions, and more. The nature of my work has depended on the nature of my client's request, the nature of my agreement with the client coupled with my own knowledge base, experience, and authority. The goal is to listen deeply and hold a space for the person who is doing the work, not to make them heal, not to cause them to heal, but to be present in a way that facilitates and supports their healing. My commitment is to discover or uncover what works for each individual client's own timing, highest good, and optimal chance of clearing an issue out all the way down to its weedy, gnarly roots. And this is an evolving process.

Recently, I have drawn inspiration from Andy Austin's approach (www.andrewtaustin.com), especially with regard to mirror box remapping. He has effected remarkable results with phantom limb pain patients. Richard Flook's meta medicine and healing (www.advancedclearingenergetics.com/about/about-richard-flook/) is of interest, Trauma Release Exercises (TRE) (www.traumaprevention.com) is an area I am interested in (other practitioners have noted its effectiveness in working with tapping and TRE in tandem, especially for those whose bodies are carrying "big" trauma as a place to start before even employing EFT). The active listening I use is along the lines of www.handinhandparenting.org, founded by the inspiring parent-child connection advocate Patty Wipfler. I draw on mindfulness and breathing exercises inspired by Dharmaseed.org, DharmapunxNYC.com, and Tarabrach.com, too.

Space precludes listing more on these energy therapy pioneers. Most of their organizations offer training and certifications.

The late Dr. Roger Callahan invented Thought Field Therapy (TFT). Visit his website at www.rogercallahan.com for more information on TFT.

Dr. Larry Nims developed the Be Set Free Fast (BSFF) method, an energy psychology. See "Tell Me About Be Set Free Fast Self-Help" for more details: www.besetfreefast.com/faq-theory.html.

Dr. John Diamond (www.drjohndiamond.com) has explored diagnosing and treating various psychological and mental problems through energy therapy.

Dr. Fred Gallo, (www.fredgallo.com) psychologist and ACEP president as of 2015, has pioneered and authored much on energy therapy.

Tapas Fleming (www.tatlife.com) developed the Tapas Acupressure Technique (TAT) for allergic reactions and clearing the impact of past traumas, gently and easily.

See my website for a more complete listing.

Online: Forums, Member Sites, Social Media, and More

Online you'll find a wealth of information about EFT, including training sites, free EFT resources, EFT social media communities, especially EFT Facebook communities, including open sites representing different organizations as well as non-affiliated EFT and/or tapping groups, professional practitioner sites, closed groups, and smaller EFT tapping circles, tapping practitioner sites, free- and paid-subscriber level member tapping sites, mega-tapping databases that publish a wide range of tapping-related material and promotions, teleseminars, online tap-related talk shows, and more.

EFT Database, Teaching Sites, and Credential-Granting Organizations

The short list is not comprehensive. It offers a few of which I know.

Emofree.com is a treasure chest of information for beginners through EFT masters. It now includes two subsites, Gold Standard

EFT and Optimal EFT (to legally share this I must say that I am a student of Gary Craig's Optimal EFT instruction found at www.optimal-eft.emofree.com). The Gold Standard site offers a comprehensive archive of three thousand case study articles on EFT applications, a free newsletter, audio and video demonstrating specific points of EFT, practitioner listings, and more. Users can obtain for free or for a donation sets of online teaching DVDs up to 120 (or more) online hours of video. The site is constantly evolving, so take your time on the site as you would with a gourmet meal or an evening with close friends. The other site, Optimal EFT, has as of this writing been offering free experiential webinars led or facilitated by Gary Craig, that concern exploring the spiritual nature of healing, including drawing on concepts such as calling in the "unseen therapist" to help work with an issue, radiating love, and more. It has been profound for me, and in the preliminary explorations with my own interested clients results have been promising.

Association for the Advancement of Meridian Energy Techniques (www.AAMET.org) Established in 1999, AAMET is the largest nonprofit international body offering consistent, effective EFT trainings, trainers and workshops listings, mentoring and support, and certified practitioners listings. Its costs are very low as all administration duties are unpaid and shared by volunteers. The website contains a plethora of useful information relating to merid- ian energy techniques and energy psychology. Recent conferences have included speakers such as Dr. Rupert Sheldrake (*The Science Delusion*, 2012), and Dr. Bradley Nelson (*The Emotion Code,* 2007).

Association for Comprehensive Energy Psychology (ACEP) (www.energypsych.org) Established in 1999, this nonprofit is AAMET's US counterpart, offering similar services through an ACEP lens, and members include the general public, EFT practitioners, and licensed mental health professionals. The offerings include conferences, seminars, including those that fulfill continuing education requirements for mental health professionals, trainings, a newsletter, practitioner listings, and more. The EFT certification track program was administered and directed by Tina Craig through December 2015, with the focus on ensuring that the practitioner has fully absorbed and can effectively practice Official and Gold Standard EFT. The training program is at the time of this writing being reorganized.

www.EFTUniverse.com was established when Gary Craig temporarily retired and gave his original site to Dawson Church Ph.D. The two are not affiliated any longer. This organization fosters and supports the EFTUniverse Levels of practitioner training. The site offers a plethora of free resources, including a newsletter, community, training certification listings, paid practitioner listings, opportunities to get involved at varying levels in the worldwide EFT community, including in a free tapping circle, videos, including tap-a-long videos, books and audio programs for sale, and more. It is also spearheading a movement to include an EFT tapping presence within the American Psychological Association.

Websites

VeteransStressProject.org Veterans with PTSD can access free EFT sessions performed by volunteer EFT practitioners who've passed field research training requirements. The project is part of a clinical study on using EFT to resolve PTSD symptoms in selected vets. So far, preliminary results are promising.

Advanced EFT Practitioner, Matrix Reimprinting practitioner, and innovator Ruthi Backenroth, MBA (www.BreakthroughRelief.com) uses EFT and other modalities as a mental exercise approach to retrain the brain and stop pain signals.

Reneé Brown (www.transformationkey.com) offers Faster and regular EFT, intuitive readings, energy healing, and more. She has been teaching and mentoring full classes and to a full schedule for for more than thirty-five years.

EFT founding master Carol Look (www.CarolLook.com) is internationally noted for her certified abundance coaching program and gratitude work. She has a regular newsletter, teaches workshops, coaches, and according to her website, uses "EFT and the Law of Attraction to clear limiting beliefs, release resistance and build prosperity consciousness." Her Abundance Store offers several guides including: Attracting Abundance with EFT, Improve Your Eyesight with EFT, and The Tapping Diet.

EFT Master Jan Luther, "the Ego Tamer," has a specialty in grief and loss (www.janluther.com) and her own creation, Ego Taming.

International trainers and husband-wife team **Alina Frank** and **Dr. Craig Weiner, DC** (www.EFTtappingtraining.com) train, mentor, and certify individuals and healing arts professionals in the art, science, and business of EFT tapping. They also moderate an active Facebook EFT tapping forum. EFT Master **Jan Luther**, "the Ego Tamer," has a specialty in grief and loss (www.janluther.com) and her own creation, Ego Taming.

Gene Monteraselli's site, www.TappingQandA.com, offers free and subscriber memberships, more than 600 articles, tap-along audios, and podcast interviews. New resources are added weekly. Check out the cool widgets "Set-up Phrase Generator" and "Tapping Ninja Videos."

Nick and **Jessica Ortner**'s juggernaut www.TheTappingSolution.com includes free access and a paid Tapping Insiders Club. The database includes articles, expert audio interviews, tapalongs, ask-the-expert podcasts, teleseminars, case studies, programs on weight release and financial abundance, and more. This brother-sister team produces the world's most widely attended online annual tapping event in the world, the annual Tapping Summit, which allows listening for a limited time for free with varying purchase options.

Nick and Jessica produced the documentary *The Tapping Solution* (2009), on a thin dime, which led to more successes, including a New York Times bestseller by the same title (2013). I am inspired by the Ortners' because the words "It's not possible" do not seem to exist even as a concept in their minds.

EFT master **Tania Prince** (www.taniaaprince.com) offers tapping, training, and inner repatterning.

Sandra Radomski addresses issues of allergies and can be found at www.allergyantidotes.com.

Kathilyn Solomon (www.EFTMinnesota.com) offers tapping, teaching on tapping, and tapping groups. The website is intended to have resources, including ebook expansions on the topics addressed herein, audios and videos, a newsletter, articles and blogs, case studies, and links to other sites. eBooks in the pipeline include subjects such as *Staying Sane With Siblings Over Holidays, Tapping On Candy-Craving Children Before Halloween, Clearing Birth Trauma, Tapping and Pregnancy, Tapping and Fertility Challenges, Targeting Bad Mom Syndrome, Clearing Shame, Exploring Ancestral Shame, Aiming Tapping at Physical Challenges, Saying Yes to Success, and more.* The podcasts address an issue from diverse expert perspectives.

Steve Wells and Dr. David Lake (www.eftdownunder.com) offer Provocative Energy Techniques (PET), which effectively "provokes" healing, and Simple Energy Techniques (SET), where people continually tap while talking about their issues.

Jondi Whitis (www.eft4results.com) is a certified AAMET EFT trainer, board member, practitioner, mentor, former Newtown trauma relief project trainer, talk-show host, East Coast TapFest annual gathering producer, and an enthusiastic supporter of what she calls EFT, "the People's Tool."

Rick Wilkes and **Cathy Vartuli**'s www.ThrivingNow.com offers free and paid level options, a newsletter, podcasts, tapping products, and more. Paid members access five live coaching calls monthly, which are recorded. Members-only forums and emails and an archived library of hundreds of recordings are available.

These two entrepreneurs blend their own tapping approaches and other techniques to address business success: **Pamela Bruner** (www.makeyoursuccessreal.com) and **Margaret Lynch** (rockstarmissionmarketing.com/rmm).

Video/Audio Podcasts

Audio and/or video podcasts include: **Gary Williams**'s www.EFTHub.Com, which interviews leaders in the tapping field. www.eftradioonline.com, produced by **Eleanore Duyndam,** offers a variety of shows hosted by EFT experts and others. www.blogtalkradio.com is another resource.

Brad Yates (www.bradyates.net and www.youtube.com/user/eftwizard) offers short tapalongs on everything from having a magnificent day to tapping in to a good night's sleep.

Community Sites

ACHPros.com (www.alternativehealthcarepros.com), founded by Karin Davidson, EFT expert and Matrix Reimprinting practitioner, has a mission statement "to unite, support, and promote alternative health care modalities and professionals by providing exceptional products, services, and information." It offers a practitioner database, workshop listings, support for EFT and many other holistic modalities, EFT training Coursebooks, and more.

EFTMastersWorldwide.com represents the EFT Founding Masters. A US-based gem with international membership, it aims to increase the reader's skill with and knowledge of EFT through articles, interviews, regularly changing videos, and workshops, listings, and links to EFT master websites. Features include Ask a Master, interviews with the masters, and Q & A from the masters.

Books

Arenson, Gloria. *Five Simple Steps to Emotional Healing.* New York: Simon and Schuster, 2001.

Bandler, Richard. *Guide to Tranceformation: How to Harness the Power of Hypnosis to Ignite Effortless and Lasting Change.* Deerfield Beach, FL: HCI, 2008.

Bandler, Richard, and John Grinder. *Frogs into Princes: Neuro Linguistic Programming.* Boulder, CO: Real People Press, 1979.

———. *The Structure of Magic, Vol. 1: A Book About Language and Therapy.* Palo Alto, CA: Science and Behavior Books, 1974.

Beer, Sue, and Emma Roberts. *Step by Step Tapping.* New York: Hachette Book Group, 2013.

Bennett, Robin Rose. The Gift of Healing Herbs. Berkeley, CA: North Atlantic Books, 2014.

Brach, Tara. *Radical Acceptance: Awakening the Love That Heals Fear and Shame.* NYC: Rider & Co., Penguin Random House, 2003.

Bruner, Pamela, and John Bulough, eds. *EFT & Beyond: Cutting Edge Techniques for Personal Transformation.* Saffron Walden, UK: Energy Publication, 2009.

Canfield, Jack, and Pamela Bruner. *Tapping Into Ultimate Success: How to Overcome Any Obstacle & Skyrocket Your Results.* Carlsbad, CA: Hay House, 2012.

Church, Dawson, PhD. *The Genie in Your Genes.* Santa Rosa, CA: Energy Psychology Press, 2009.

Diamond, John, MD. *Life Energy: Using the Meridians to Unlock the Hidden Power of Your Emotions.* St. Paul, MN: Paragon House, 1990.

Feinstein, David, Donna Eden, and Gary Craig. *The Promise of Energy Psychology: Revolutionary Tools for Dramatic Personal Change.* New York: Jeremy P. Tarcher/Penguin, 2005.

Fone, Helena. *Emotional Freedom Technique for Dummies.* West Sussex, UK: For Dummies, 2008.

Gallo, Fred, PhD, ed. *Energy Psychology in Psychotherapy: A Comprehensive Sourcebook.* New York: Norton, 2002.

Gallo, Fred PhD, and Harry Vincenzi, EDD. *Energy Tapping: How to Rapidly Eliminate Anxiety, Depression, Cravings, and More Using Energy Psychology.* Oakland, CA: New Harbinger Publications, Inc. 2008.

Heller, Steven, and Terry Lee Steele. *Monsters & Magical Sticks: There's No Such Thing as Hypnosis?* Tempe, AZ: Original Falcon Press, 2009.

Levine, Peter A. PhD. *In an Unspoken Voice: How the Body Releases Trauma and Restores Goodness.* Lyons, CO: ERGOS Institute Press, 2010.

———. *Waking the Tiger: Healing Trauma.* Berkeley, CA: North Atlantic Press, 1997.

Look, Carol. *Attracting Abundance with EFT.* Coeur D'Alene, ID: Crown Media & Printing, 2008.

Luther, Jan. *Grief Is Mourning Sickness: What to Expect When You Are Grieving and What to Do About It.* Charlotte, NC: TRS Press, 2012.

Maté, Gabor, MD. *In the Realm of the Hungry Ghosts: Close Encounters With Addictions.* Berkeley, CA: North Atlantic Books, 2010.

Miller, Deborah D., PhD. *The Dragon with the Flames of Love: Helping Children with Serious Illness Improve the Quality of Their Lives.* Ashland, KY: Light Within Enterprises, 2014.

Ortner, Jessica. *The Tapping Solution for Weight Loss & Body Confidence: A Woman's Guide to Stressing Less, Weighing Less, and Loving More.* Carlsbad, CA: Hay House, 2014.

Ortner, Nick. *The Tapping Solution: A Revolutionary System for Stress-Free Living.* Carlsbad, CA: Hay House, 2013.

Temes, Roberta, PhD. *Tapping Cure.* Cambridge, MA: Capo Press, 2006.

Siegel, Daniel J., MD. Brainstorm. *The Power and Purpose of the Teenage Brain.* New York: Jeremy P. Tarcher/Penguin, 2013.

Wells, Steve, and David Lake, MD. *Emotional Healing With Provocative Energy Techniques.* DVD. Sydney, AU, 2014.

———. *Enjoy Emotional Freedom: Simple Techniques for Living Life to the Full.* Downers Grove, IL: Inter-Varsity Press, 2010.

Wipfler, Patty. *Parenting Pamphlets—Parenting by Connection: Listening Effectively to Children.* Palo Alto, CA: Hand in Hand Parenting, 2006. (Any podcasts, articles, or listserves from the Parenting by Connection nonprofit on YouTube or the website handinhand.org.)

Vajda, Debby. "Online Energy Therapy Bibliography." www.the4dgroup.com/DebbyVajda/bibliography.htm.

GET MORE AT LLEWELLYN.COM

Visit us online to browse hundreds of our books and decks, plus sign up to receive our e-newsletters and exclusive online offers.

- Free tarot readings • Spell-a-Day • Moon phases
- Recipes, spells, and tips • Blogs • Encyclopedia
- Author interviews, articles, and upcoming events

GET SOCIAL WITH LLEWELLYN

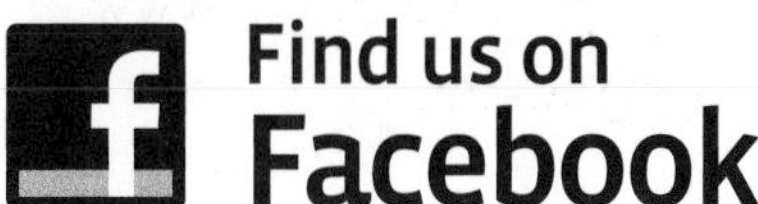

www.Facebook.com/LlewellynBooks

Follow us on twitter™

www.Twitter.com/Llewellynbooks

GET BOOKS AT LLEWELLYN

LLEWELLYN ORDERING INFORMATION

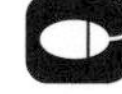

Order online: Visit our website at www.llewellyn.com to select your books and place an order on our secure server.

Order by phone:
- Call toll free within the U.S. at 1-877-NEW-WRLD (1-877-639-9753)
- Call toll free within Canada at 1-866-NEW-WRLD (1-866-639-9753)
- We accept VISA, MasterCard, and American Express

Order by mail:
Send the full price of your order (MN residents add 6.875% sales tax) in U.S. funds, plus postage and handling to: Llewellyn Worldwide, 2143 Wooddale Drive
Woodbury, MN 55125-2989

POSTAGE AND HANDLING

STANDARD (U.S. & Canada):
(Please allow 12 business days)
$25.00 and under, add $4.00.
$25.01 and over, FREE SHIPPING.

INTERNATIONAL ORDERS (airmail only):
$16.00 for one book, plus $3.00 for each additional book.

Visit us online for more shipping options. Prices subject to change.

FREE CATALOG!

To order, call 1-877-NEW-WRLD ext. 8236 or visit our website

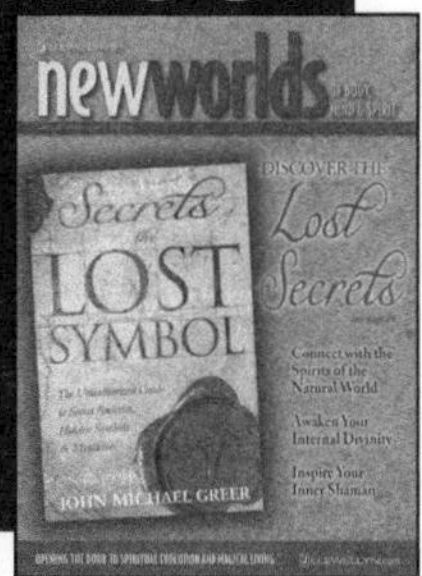

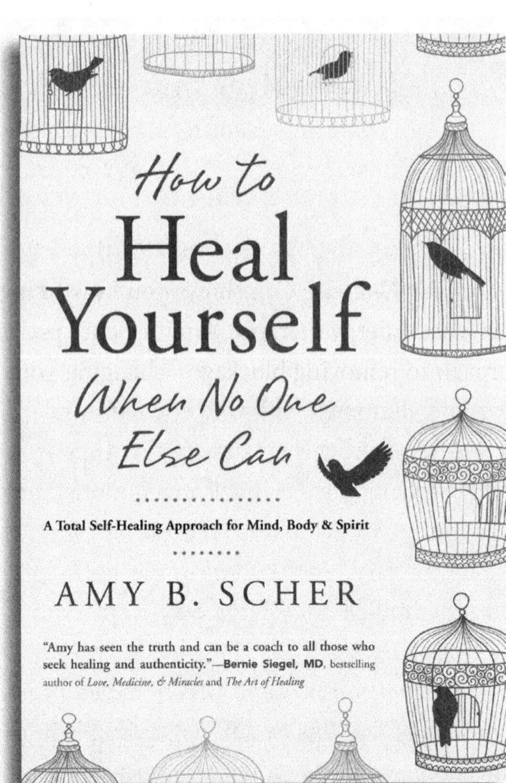
How to
Heal
Yourself
When No One
Else Can
A Total Self-Healing Approach for Mind, Body & Spirit
AMY B. SCHER
"Amy has seen the truth and can be a coach to all those who seek healing and authenticity."—Bernie Siegel, MD, bestselling author of Love, Medicine, & Miracles and The Art of Healing

How to Heal Yourself When No One Else Can

A Total Self-Healing Approach for Mind, Body, and Spirit

AMY B. SCHER

Using energy therapy and emotional healing techniques, *How to Heal Yourself When No One Else Can* shows you how to love, accept, and be yourself no matter what. Energy therapist Amy B. Scher presents a down-to-earth three-part approach to removing blockages, changing your relationship with stress, and coming into alignment with who you truly are.

After overcoming late-stage chronic Lyme disease, Amy came to an important epiphany that healing is much more than just physical. Her dramatic story of healing serves as a powerful example of how beneficial it is to address our emotional energies, particularly when nothing else works. Discover the four main areas of imbalance and the easy ways to address them on your journey to complete and permanent healing. With Amy's guidance, you can get rid of blocks you never knew you had and finally move forward. Whether you are experiencing physical symptoms or are just feeling lost, sad, anxious, or emotionally unbalanced, this book can improve your wellbeing and your life.

978-0-7387-4554-1, 288 pp., 6 x 9, $17.99

To order, call 1-877-NEW-WRLD

Prices subject to change without notice

Order at Llewellyn.com 24 hours a day, 7 days a week

DELLA TEMPLE

Tame Your Inner Critic

Find Peace & Contentment to Live Your Life on Purpose